Future Healthcare 2050

Future Healthcare 2050

How Artificial Intelligence Transforms the Patient-Physician Journey

Barry P. Chaiken, MD

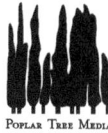

POPLAR TREE MEDIA

Poplar Tree Media
Boston

Barry P. Chaiken, MD
Poplar Tree Media
14 Durham Street
Boston MA 02115-5301
barrychaiken.com
bchaiken@docsnetwork.com

Book Design by Barry P. Chaiken, MD

Hardcover (Print of Demand) ISBN: 978-1-7367021-5-4
eBook ISBN: 978-1-7367021-4-7
Library of Congress Catalog Control Number: 2024952914

To the courageous journalists around the world who risk their lives seeking and reporting the truth and facts, safeguarding democracy and the freedoms that uphold our life, liberty, and the pursuit of happiness.

Contents

CHAPTER 1

A Journey to Healthcare AI: Quality, Technology, and the Promise of AI

In the early 1980s, sitting in Dr. Heather Palmer's classroom at the Harvard School of Public Health, I had no idea that my journey in healthcare quality would eventually lead me to artificial intelligence (AI). Back then, the very idea of measuring healthcare quality was revolutionary—even controversial. Doctors were unquestioned authorities, healthcare was measured in volume rather than value, and our most sophisticated analytical tool was a handheld calculator. But Dr. Palmer's passionate conviction that *you can't manage what you can't measure* would prove prophetic in ways none of us could have imagined.

As an Epidemic Intelligence Service (EIS) officer stationed at the Allegheny County Health Department in Pittsburgh, I faced my first real test of Dr. Palmer's measurement principle during a food poisoning investigation. EIS officers are Centers for Disease Control and Prevention (CDC) employees and first responders when disease outbreaks occur. Armed with completed questionnaires and a handheld calculator, I spent eight painstaking hours creating food-borne attack-rate tables on paper spreadsheets. Each calculation had to be double-checked, and each entry had to be meticulously verified.

During a later training visit to the CDC in Atlanta, I first glimpsed the future—a personal computer. The potential was obvious, and my natural curiosity took over. I soon purchased my first-generation IBM PC, eager to explore its capabilities. When I later handled a measles outbreak investigation for the New Jersey State Department of Health, I had to get special permission and reserve time to use their single PC in the MIS department. But that one computer transformed what would have been days of manual calculations into a manageable task.

My curiosity about technology's potential became a driving force in my career. As technology evolved, I was drawn to learning each new advancement, always asking: How can this improve healthcare? More importantly, I discovered my calling as a bridge between two worlds—able to translate between healthcare professionals and technology experts, helping each understand the other's perspective.

My first venture into healthcare technology came at a startup where we saw an opportunity that others had missed. While most physicians still wrote their clinical notes, we envisioned using Microsoft Word templates with pull-down menus to streamline documentation. It seems obvious now, but simply using computers to facilitate clinical documentation was revolutionary in those early days. Working alongside medical specialists to create these templates taught me my first crucial lesson about healthcare technology: success requires a deep understanding of clinical workflow and technology.

This belief in technology's potential to transform healthcare led me to collaborate with Dr. Larry Weed, a visionary who had already revolutionized medical documentation with his *problem-oriented medical record* and *SOAP* note format. Dr. Weed's *Problem*

Knowledge Coupler was ahead of its time—it used computer logic to generate differential diagnoses based on signs and symptoms, an early predecessor to today's AI diagnostic tools.

These experiences revealed another truth: healthcare is an incredibly complex ecosystem that few technologists genuinely understand. From medical terminology to insurance pre-authorizations, from licensing requirements to payment systems—each aspect requires careful translation between the clinical and technical worlds.

My work with Dr. Weed reinforced something crucial: technology is not just about efficiency but improving quality and safety in healthcare. However, I confronted healthcare's harsh economic realities as I moved into roles with companies developing software for healthcare providers. In an era of spiraling costs, decision-makers had three primary questions about any new technology: Will it save money? Will it generate revenue? Will it reduce staffing costs? Quality and safety improvements, however necessary, were often viewed as secondary benefits.

Yet I believed there was always a *third way* to meausre benefits—a more profound analysis that could reveal hidden value. My background in economics taught me about externalities—those hidden costs and benefits that do not appear in immediate calculations and are found only through open-minded thinking. Preventing an unnecessary test or procedure does not just save its cost; it saves downstream costs from potential complications, reduces patient stress and lost work time, and frees up medical resources for essential care. Finding these hidden connections became my specialty—asking the right questions to understand how technology could serve quality and financial goals simultaneously.

My commitment to healthcare quality led me to pursue certification in the field, but this was just the beginning. Soon, I found myself learning and teaching—sharing my unique perspective on information technology with future quality professionals. The experience of writing certification exam questions, after extensive training by the National Board of Medical Examiners, taught me something crucial: quality is not just about having standards but how you measure and evaluate them. Just as I had learned from Dr. Palmer years before, *you can't manage what you can't measure*, and you can't measure without the right tools and the correct data.

As I moved through roles as a lecturer, chairperson of the continuing medical education committee, and eventually board member, I watched healthcare's relationship with technology evolve. The handheld calculators of my early days had given way to sophisticated software systems, yet the fundamental questions remained: How do we measure quality? How do we improve it? How do we prove we are making a difference?

After decades of working with healthcare technology, I see it as a flower garden. Each new technology, like a flower, can appear beautiful and full of promise. Some technologies bring precisely what they promise—efficiency, improved care, and better outcomes. Despite their allure, others prove toxic to an organization if not carefully chosen and properly cultivated. I witnessed the consequences of both scenarios: hospitals rushing to implement electronic health record systems without evaluating workflows or adequately training staff, essentially digitizing broken processes, and sometimes even causing patient harm. I have seen expensive technology solutions wither unused, draining resources that could have nourished other improvements.

However, I have also seen organizations that took the time to prepare their soil—carefully evaluating their processes, training their staff, and understanding the entire care ecosystem before planting new technology. These organizations reaped rich harvests of improved efficiency, better patient outcomes, and enhanced staff satisfaction.

Now, as we stand at the beginning of the AI era in healthcare, these lessons have never been more critical. AI is the most alluring flower yet in healthcare's technology garden—promising unprec-edented diagnostic, treatment planning, and quality improvement capabilities. But like any powerful tool, its successful cultivation will require wisdom gained from past experiences, careful attention to process and people, and a deep understanding of its potential and dangers.

In the following chapters, we will explore how to cultivate AI in healthcare's garden—choosing the right applications, preparing the ground for successful implementation, and nurturing imple-mentations that truly improve care.

As we embark on this exploration of healthcare AI, I leave you with the most crucial lessons from my journey: Listen—truly listen—to all stakeholders, understanding what change means for each of them. Never take shortcuts in planning; embrace change management as your closest ally. When evaluating any new tech-nology, especially AI, carefully weigh benefits and risks from every perspective. Be thorough in calculating costs and actual benefits, documenting everything in detail. Most importantly, let the facts, not enthusiasm or fear, guide your decisions. And remember: whether you are leading the charge or supporting those who are, healthcare's transformation through AI will require bold leadership and strong contributors working together.

The chapters ahead will show you how to apply these lessons to the most potent technology healthcare has yet encountered. The garden of artificial intelligence holds infinite promise—but only if we cultivate it wisely.

Before we explore AI in healthcare, let me explain how this book is designed to guide you through this transformative journey. Throughout this book, you will find three distinct features that enrich your exploration: *Historical Context* sections that root our discussion in real-world experience and show how past innovations inform future discoveries, *Sidebars* that spotlight crucial concepts deserving special attention, and *Bedside Consults* drawn from my blog that offer practical, real-world insights.

To support your healthcare AI journey, a comprehensive *Glossary* helps demystify technical terms and concepts, ensuring you can confidently navigate healthcare and technology discussions. Each chapter includes carefully curated *Endnotes* providing context and source materials. For easy access, you will find a QR code in the *Endnotes* section that links to a dedicated webpage where all source materials are available with live URL links. This interconnected approach ensures you have both the context you need within the book and seamless access to a deeper exploration of topics that interest you.

Timeline of Transformative Innovation

1700

1747   Dr. James Lind conducts the first clinical trial
1761   Dr. Leopold Auenbrugger introduces percussion as a diagnostic technique
1785   Edward Cartwright invents the power loom

1800

1816   Dr. René Laennec invents the stethoscope
1847   Dr. Ignaz Semmelweis discovers handwashing reduces mortality
1855   Florence Nightingale pioneers statistical analysis to predict and prevent hospital deaths
1894   Herman Hollerith builds the first electromechanical punched-card machine

1900 – 1949

1904   Dr. Ernest Codman tracks patient outcomes
1905   First electrocardiogram transmitted remotely by Dr. Willem Einthoven
1906   Santiago Ramón y Cajal reveals neuron communication mechanisms
1911   Frederick Winslow Taylor applies engineering principles to improve industrial processes
1913   Henry Ford introduces assembly line manufacturing

1919   AT&T implements first automatic telephone switching system

1924   Sidney Pressey invents a mechanical teaching machine

1928   Justice Louis Brandeis establishes the principles of privacy law

1938   Orson Welles broadcasts *War of the Worlds*

1941   Dr. Howard Florey and Ernst Chain successfully test the first human use of penicillin

1942   J. Robert Oppenheimer leads the Manhattan Project

1943   Dr. Warren McCulloch and Walter Pitts lay the foundation for neural networks

1943   Cryptographers at Britain's Bletchly Park demonstrate how mathematical techniques could protect sensitive information

1945   Vannevar Bush imagines modern information systems

1948   Framingham Heart Study begins

1948   Claude Shannon revolutionizes information theory

1950 – 1969

1950   Alan Turing proposes the *Turing Test*

1952   Bell Labs builds *Audrey*, the first speech recognition system

1953   Taiichi Ohno creates Toyota's production system

1954   Paul Meehl demonstrates how statistical methods could complement clinical judgment

1954   Dr. Homer Warner builds the first clinical decision support system

1956   *Logic Theorist* becomes the first AI program

1956   Leonard Skeggs develops an automated blood analyzer

1957   Frank Rosenblatt develops the *perceptron*, the first artificial neural network

1958   Thalidomide prescribed to pregnant women in the UK leads to congenital disabilities

1962   Dr. Morris Collen pioneers the first automated medical history system

1965   U.S. Postal Service implements OCR

1969   The U.S. Department of Defense introduces APRANET, the precursor to the internet

1970 -

1970   NASA rescues Apollo XIII

1972   Hewlett Packard releases the HP-35, the first scientific pocket calculator

1976   Dr. Edward Shortliffe introduces *MYCIN*, the first expert system in medicine

1976   Joseph Weizenbaum critiques over-reliance on computers

1976   National swine flu vaccination program leads to unexpected cases of Guillain-Barré syndrome

1979   Three Mile Island Nuclear Generating Station meltdown

1980   Diagnosis-Related Groups (DRGs) implemented

1982   Tylenol bottle tampering tragedy

1986   Lawrence Rabiner revolutionizes speech recognition

1991   Unified Medical Language System (UMLS) released

1994   Dr. Ken Kizer transforms the Veterans Health Administration

Part I

Understanding Tomorrow's Healthcare: AI Foundations

The promise of artificial intelligence (AI) in healthcare represents one of the most profound shifts in modern medicine, akin to the advent of antibiotics or the discovery of DNA's double helix. As a public health physician specializing in healthcare information technology and AI, I have witnessed firsthand how this transformation extends far beyond automating routine tasks—it represents a fundamental reimagining of how we deliver, manage, and improve patient care. Through my work with healthcare organizations nationwide, I have seen the tremendous potential and risks of implementing AI in healthcare settings.

At its core, AI empowers healthcare professionals to transcend the limitations of current methods. By leveraging vast amounts of data—from imaging and genomics to electronic health records and real-time monitoring—AI systems can reveal insights that often remain hidden in the complexity of medical data. These tools are not about replacing clinicians but augmenting their expertise, providing support that sharpens decision-making and frees up time for the human interaction that patients value most. Whether detecting subtle patterns in diagnostic scans or tailoring interventions to individual patients, AI helps bridge the gap between precision and personalization in care delivery, offering a new frontier of possibilities.

In the following chapters, we explore the intricate interplay of technology, innovation, and human expertise in transforming healthcare. We begin with the fundamentals of healthcare AI, examining the technical foundations and the ethical imperatives that must guide its implementation. This foundation is crucial for healthcare leaders and professionals to make informed decisions about AI adoption while ensuring equitable and responsible deployment.

We then delve into the fascinating world of multimodal AI, showing how combining different data types—from medical imaging to clinical notes—provides deeper insights and more accurate clinical decision support. We follow by exploring how AI and predictive analytics work in synergy, enabling healthcare systems to shift from reactive to proactive care delivery models. The real-world applications range from ensuring proper staffing in anticipation of patient surges to preventing equipment downtime through predictive maintenance.

My narrative then transitions to AI's practical role in healthcare delivery, examining how these technologies enhance clinical judgment while ensuring patient care remains grounded in empathy and trust. We explore how AI augments human expertise rather than replacing it, maintaining the essential human elements of healthcare delivery. A dedicated chapter on virtual assistants demonstrates how these tools revolutionize patient interaction and administrative processes, enabling healthcare providers to focus more on direct patient care.

Throughout these chapters, I combine theoretical understanding with practical insights from real-world implementations. Drawing from my experience helping healthcare organizations navigate this complex landscape, I address the technical aspects of AI and the strategic considerations, change management requirements, and ethical implications that healthcare leaders must navigate.

I wrote this book for healthcare executives, clinical leaders, technology decision-makers, and anyone interested in learning about the potential of healthcare AI. Whether you are just beginning to explore AI implementation or looking to optimize existing AI initiatives, these chapters provide the strategic framework and practical insights needed to move forward effectively. I pay special attention to ensuring AI applications help bridge healthcare disparities, particularly in underserved communities, where technology can extend the reach and improve the quality of care delivery.

As we embrace these advancements, our focus remains clear: leveraging technology to improve lives while honoring the principles of compassion, equity, and excellence that define the practice of medicine. The transformative potential of AI in healthcare is immense—I have seen it firsthand. However, realizing this potential requires careful planning, strategic implementation, and a clear understanding of opportunities and challenges.

I invite you to join me as we explore how artificial intelligence can help us build a more efficient, effective, and equitable healthcare system for all.

CHAPTER 2

Fundamentals of Healthcare AI

In 1950, Alan Turing asked, "Can machines think? His groundbreaking paper "Computing Machinery and Intelligence" laid the foundation for artificial intelligence (AI), proposing what would become known as the *Turing Test*. As Turing envisioned machines that could mimic human intelligence, early medical pioneers like Dr. Homer Warner at LDS Hospital began exploring computer-aided medical decision-making in the 1950s. These first steps toward combining computing power with healthcare expertise marked the beginning of a journey that continues to transform medicine today.

Healthcare has evolved through technological innovation—from the stethoscope revolutionizing physical examination to magnetic resonance imaging transforming diagnostic capabilities. Today, AI and machine learning (ML) promise a similar transformative potential, inspiring us to push the boundaries of what is possible in healthcare. Unlike previous innovations that extended human capabilities, AI represents something fundamentally different: systems that learn and adapt based on experience.

These sophisticated tools promise to revolutionize everything from patient care and clinical decision-making to medical research and administrative efficiency. To effectively harness this potential, healthcare professionals must empower themselves with a deep understanding of the fundamental concepts underlying AI and its applications in healthcare settings.

At its core, AI refers to computer systems capable of performing tasks that typically require human intelligence. These tasks include visual perception, speech recognition, decision-making, and natural language processing. ML, a subset of AI, focuses on developing algorithms that enable computer systems to learn and improve their performance without explicit programming. Instead, these systems learn from patterns in data, making them valuable in healthcare, where vast amounts of complex patient data exist.

The successful implementation of healthcare AI hinges on three critical pillars: high-quality data, sophisticated algorithms, and robust validation processes. Healthcare data, in its various forms, directly influences the performance and reliability of AI systems. Issues such as data quality, biased datasets, and the misrepresentation of diverse patient populations lead to suboptimal AI performance or even perpetuate existing healthcare disparities.

Training the Machine

In 1957, Frank Rosenblatt developed the *perceptron*, the first artificial neural network capable of learning from examples. This breakthrough at Cornell Aeronautical Laboratory parallels modern healthcare ML systems' ability to learn from patient data. Just as Rosenblatt's perceptron learned to recognize simple patterns, today's healthcare algorithms learn to identify complex medical patterns across vast datasets.

Healthcare ML algorithms generally fall into three main categories: supervised learning, unsupervised learning, and reinforcement learning. Supervised learning, the most common approach, involves training algorithms on labeled data where the desired output is known. For example, training an algorithm to identify diabetic retinopathy in retinal images requires a dataset of images that medical experts have labeled as either showing signs of the condition or not.

Unsupervised learning algorithms, in contrast, work with unlabeled data to discover hidden patterns or groupings. These algorithms excel at tasks like patient segmentation or identifying unusual patterns in medical data that might indicate emerging health trends or rare conditions.

The third category, reinforcement learning, involves algorithms that learn optimal actions through trial and error, receiving feedback as rewards or penalties. This approach shows promise in treatment optimization and clinical trial design.

Natural language processing, another crucial component of healthcare AI, focuses on the interaction between computers and human language. It enables the extraction of valuable information from unstructured clinical notes, medical literature, and patient reports. This capability is invaluable for automated medical coding, clinical decision support, and monitoring of adverse drug events.

The success of healthcare AI heavily depends on the ability to reduce statistical bias and error in predictions. Traditional statistical methods often need help with the complexity and volume of healthcare data, but ML approaches address these challenges through several mechanisms.

Large-scale data analysis can identify subtle patterns that conventional methods might miss. Additionally, advanced techniques such as regularization and cross-validation help ensure that

AI models remain robust and generalizable across different patient populations.

Implementing healthcare AI requires careful attention to the challenges of cross-domain generalization. This concept becomes important when deploying AI systems across healthcare institutions, patient populations, or geographical regions. An AI model trained on data from one hospital might perform differently when deployed in another due to variations in patient demographics, clinical practices, or equipment availability. To address these challenges, healthcare organizations increasingly turn to federated learning.

Sidebar: Federated Learning

Google researchers introduced *federated learning* in 2017, proposing a revolutionary approach to distributed machine learning that preserved data privacy. This innovation emerged during a period of increasing concern about data protection, where Health Insurance Portability and Accountability Act (HIPAA) privacy regulations and international privacy laws were shaping the landscape of health data sharing.

Federated learning represents a significant advancement in AI development. It allows institutions to collaborate on AI models while maintaining patient privacy. This approach enables multiple healthcare organizations to contribute to model development without directly sharing sensitive patient data, addressing critical privacy and regulatory concerns.

The core mechanism involves each participating institution maintaining its local dataset and training a local version of the model. These institutions then share only the model parameters with a central server, aggregating them to create an improved global model. This global model is then redistributed to all participating institutions, creating a continuous improvement cycle while preserving data privacy.

Real-world applications of federated learning have already emerged. For instance, the *MELLODDY* project demonstrates its potential in drug discovery, enabling collaboration among pharmaceutical companies without sharing proprietary data. Similarly, the *HealthChain* project showcases how federated learning supports secure AI model development across multiple healthcare institutions for applications ranging from medical imaging to precision medicine. These examples highlight the diverse ways in which federated learning can be applied.

However, implementing federated learning settings presents several challenges. For example, data heterogeneity across institutions leads to biased or poorly calibrated global models. The frequent communication required for federated learning between local institutions and the central server creates significant computational overhead. Aggregating model parameters from multiple sources makes it more difficult to interpret and explain the resulting AI models, a crucial consideration in healthcare applications.

To address these challenges, healthcare organizations need to implement specific best practices. These include establishing common data standards and protocols to ensure consistency across institutions, implementing secure aggregation protocols to protect privacy during parameter sharing, and developing robust validation processes to ensure model accuracy and fairness across different patient populations. Clear governance frameworks and data-sharing agreements are essential to align incentives and maintain transparency among participating institutions. In addition, participating institutions must sort out the model's intellectual property rights and document them in participation agreements to ensure that any financial gains from its use are distributed equitably.

Despite the challenges, federated learning can significantly advance healthcare AI while safeguarding patient privacy. As the technology matures, it will enable more collaborative, efficient, and privacy-preserving approaches to AI development, ultimately supporting more personalized and equitable patient care.

Model Training

In 1943, Dr. Warren McCulloch and Walter Pitts published their groundbreaking paper on neural networks, "A Logical Calculus of Ideas Immanent in Nervous Activity." Their work, modeling how biological neurons might perform computational tasks, laid the foundation for modern neural network training. While far more sophisticated, today's healthcare AI training processes still reflect their fundamental insight about the importance of carefully structured model training.

The training process for healthcare AI models requires rigorous attention to detail and validation. This process begins with the careful selection and preparation of training data. Healthcare data often contains inherent biases, missing values, and inconsistencies that developers must address before training can begin. Data preprocessing steps include:

- Normalization of laboratory values.
- Handling of missing data.
- Careful consideration of potential biases in the training dataset.

During training, developers need to regularly evaluate models using appropriate performance metrics. In healthcare applications, these metrics extend beyond simple accuracy measures, including sensitivity, specificity, and positive predictive value. The choice of evaluation metrics should align with the clinical context and potential consequences of model errors. For instance, in cancer screening applications, high sensitivity (minimizing false negatives) might be prioritized over high specificity (minimizing false positives).

Model interpretability is particularly important in healthcare applications. While some ML models, especially deep learning networks, can achieve impressive performance, they often operate as *black boxes*, making it difficult to understand how they arrive at their predictions. This lack of transparency presents challenges where clinicians must understand and trust the basis for AI-generated recommendations. Various techniques for improving model interpretability have emerged, including attention mechanisms, feature importance analysis, and developing more inherently interpretable model architectures.

Statistical bias and error reduction remain critical challenges for healthcare AI. ML approaches help address these challenges through several mechanisms. Representative sampling ensures that training data reflects the target population, reducing selection bias. Feature selection algorithms automatically identify the most relevant variables for predictions, minimizing omitted variable bias. Regularization techniques prevent overfitting by penalizing unnecessarily complex models, while cross-validation methods assess model performance on independent test sets.

The development of healthcare AI systems requires considering the importance of continuous learning and adaptation. Unlike traditional medical devices or diagnostic tools, AI systems improve their performance over time as they encounter new data. However, this capability introduces additional complexity regarding validation and regulatory compliance. Healthcare organizations should establish robust processes for monitoring model performance, detecting potential degradation or drift, and updating models while maintaining their safety and effectiveness.

Fairness, Accountability, and Transparency

In 1976, computer scientist Joseph Weizenbaum published "Computer Power and Human Reason," warning about over-reliance on computer decision-making in sensitive domains. His experience with *ELIZA*, an early natural language processing program that could simulate a psychotherapist, led him to advocate for maintaining human judgment in critical decisions. This prescient concern mirrors modern discussions about AI accountability and transparency.

Ensuring the ethical implementation of AI requires careful consideration of fairness, accountability, and transparency. AI systems need to be designed and validated to perform equitably across different patient populations, avoiding discrimination based on many factors, including race, gender, or socioeconomic status. This requires careful attention to potential biases in training data and regular monitoring of model performance across different demographic groups.

The integration of AI systems into clinical workflows presents another significant challenge. Healthcare professionals must receive training to effectively use and interpret AI outputs, understanding their capabilities and limitations. The goal is not to replace human clinical judgment but to augment it with AI-generated insights and recommendations. This requires careful attention to appropriate documentation of AI-assisted decision-making, clear communication of model confidence levels, and construction of clinical workflows that limit automation bias.

It is essential that organizations also consider ongoing maintenance and update requirements when deploying healthcare AI. This maintenance includes monitoring model performance, retraining with new data when necessary, and maintaining the technical infrastructure required to support AI operations. Organizations should also establish clear protocols for handling edge cases or situations where AI systems produce unexpected or incorrect results.

Implementing AI requires robust data management and processing infrastructure. This includes data collection, storage, preprocessing systems, and computing resources capable of training and running complex AI models. Organizations also need to implement appropriate security measures to protect sensitive patient data throughout the AI pipeline.

Organizations should carefully inspect vendor healthcare AI systems to distinguish between actual AI applications and simpler rule-based expert systems. Many tools marketed as AI solutions are expert systems driven by predefined rules and algorithms. While these systems are valuable, they need adaptability and learning capabilities to be considered an AI system.

As I look to the future, several trends will likely shape healthcare AI's evolution. The continued development of more sophisticated algorithms, including deep learning and neural network advances, will enable AI systems to tackle increasingly complex healthcare tasks. Improvements in model interpretability and fairness will address current limitations and concerns. The growing availability of high-quality healthcare data and advances in computing power and infrastructure will enable more powerful and sophisticated AI applications.

Ultimately, the successful implementation of AI in healthcare requires a balanced approach that combines technical sophistication with practical considerations and ethical principles. Organizations must invest in appropriate infrastructure, establish robust validation processes, and ensure their AI systems perform equitably across diverse patient populations. Most importantly, they need to maintain a clear focus on the ultimate goal: improving patient care and outcomes through the responsible application of AI technology.

While understanding healthcare AI's technical foundations and implementation challenges is crucial, the ethical frameworks that guide its use are equally important. My *Bedside Consult* examines these ethical considerations through the lens of large language models (LLMs), representing one of healthcare AI's most rapidly evolving areas.

Bedside Consult: Charting an Ethical AI Course— The LLM Challenge in Healthcare

As LLMs continue to make significant inroads into healthcare, we find ourselves at a critical juncture. The potential benefits of these AI systems are immense, but so too are the ethical challenges they present. To navigate this complex landscape, we need a robust ethical framework to guide the development, deployment, and use of LLMs in medicine. This bioethical framework is grounded in four fundamental principles: beneficence, non-maleficence, autonomy, and justice. By examining these principles in the context of LLMs, we can better understand how to harness the power of AI while upholding the core values of medical ethics.

Beneficence: Maximizing the Potential of LLMs

The principle of beneficence calls on us to act in patients' best interests and maximize potential benefits. In the context of LLMs, this principle challenges us to fully leverage these technologies to improve patient outcomes, enhance clinical decision-making, and advance medical research. For instance, LLMs analyze vast amounts of medical literature and patient data to suggest personalized treatment plans or identify rare diseases that human clinicians might overlook. However, realizing these benefits requires careful implementation and continuous evaluation to ensure that LLMs contribute positively to patient care.

Non-maleficence: Safeguarding Against Harm

Non-maleficence, the principle of *doing no harm*, is particularly crucial when dealing with robust AI systems like LLMs. The potential for harm exists in various forms, from misdiagnosis due to biased or incorrect outputs to patient privacy breaches. One significant concern is the phenomenon of *hallucinations*, where LLMs generate plausible-sounding but factually inaccurate information. In a medical context, such errors could have severe consequences. To uphold non-maleficence, we must implement robust safety measures, including rigorous testing, continuous monitoring, and clear protocols for human oversight of AI-generated recommendations. Creating proper workflows to ensure adequate human oversight remains challenging in clinical settings due to the need to integrate AI tools into existing electronic health records properly.

Autonomy: Empowering Patients and Clinicians

Respect for autonomy is a cornerstone of medical ethics, emphasizing the right of patients to make informed decisions about their care. In the era of LLMs, preserving autonomy becomes more complex. On one hand, LLMs enhance patient autonomy by providing access to vast amounts of medical information and personalized health insights. On the other hand, there is a risk of overreliance on AI, diminishing the role of human judgment in medical decision-making. Striking the right balance requires transparent communication about using LLMs in patient care and ensuring that patients and clinicians understand the capabilities and limitations of these AI systems.

Justice: Ensuring Equitable Access and Outcomes

The principle of justice in healthcare calls for a fair distribution of benefits and risks. As LLMs become more prevalent in medicine, we must ensure their benefits are accessible to all patient populations and not exacerbate existing healthcare disparities. This involves addressing bias in training data, ensuring diverse representation in AI development teams, and considering the global implications of LLM deployment. Moreover, we need to be vigilant about the potential for LLMs to perpetuate or amplify societal biases that could lead to discriminatory healthcare outcomes.

To illustrate how these bioethical principles apply in real-world scenarios, let us consider two hypothetical case studies:

Case Study 1: The AI-Assisted Diagnosis

In this scenario, an LLM-powered diagnostic tool suggests a rare condition the attending physician had not considered. The healthcare AI bases its recommendation on a complex analysis of the patient's symptoms, medical history, and recent medical literature. However, pursuing this diagnosis would require invasive and expensive tests.

This case touches on all four bioethical principles. Beneficence and non-maleficence are at play in weighing the potential benefit of identifying a rare condition against the risks and discomfort of additional testing. Autonomy comes into focus when considering how to communicate this AI-generated suggestion to the patient and involve them in decision-making. Justice arises regarding resource allocation and whether such AI tools are equitably available to all patients.

Case Study 2: The LLM-Generated Treatment Plan

In another scenario, an oncologist uses an LLM to generate a personalized treatment plan for a cancer patient. The AI suggests an experimental therapy that has shown promise in recent clinical trials but is not yet the standard of care. The LLM's recommendation is based on an analysis of the patient's genetic profile and the latest research data.

This case highlights the tension between innovation and established medical practice. Beneficence drives the pursuit of more effective treatments, while non-maleficence urges caution with unproven therapies. Respecting patient autonomy requires carefully explaining the AI's role in generating this recommendation and the uncertainties involved. Justice considerations arise regarding access to such cutting-edge AI tools and experimental treatments and the ability to pay for them.

The Path Forward: A Collaborative Approach

As we navigate these complex ethical landscapes, it becomes clear that the most effective use of LLMs will be through a collaborative approach. Patients should be transparent about using AI tools and sharing results and insights with their clinicians. Healthcare providers, in turn, must be open about using LLMs in patient care, explaining how these tools inform their decision-making process.

This collaborative model aligns with the bioethical principles we have discussed. It respects patient autonomy by involving them in the AI-augmented care process. It promotes beneficence by combining the analytical power of LLMs with human clinicians' experiential knowledge and empathy. It supports non-maleficence by creating multiple checkpoints to catch potential errors or biases. It also advances justice by fostering a transparent system where AI is open to scrutiny and improvement.

A Call to Action: Shaping an Ethical Future for AI in Medicine

As we stand on the brink of a new era in healthcare, shaped by the transformative potential of LLMs and other AI technologies, we all have a role to play in ensuring that this future aligns with our ethical values.

> **To healthcare leaders and policymakers**: invest in developing ethical guidelines and governance structures for AI in medicine.

> **To clinicians**: embrace these new tools while maintaining critical judgment and empathetic care.

> **To patients**: engage actively in your healthcare, asking questions about how AI is used in your care and sharing your experiences with AI health tools.

> **To developers of LLMs and other healthcare AI**: embed ethical considerations into every stage of your design and development process. Seek diverse perspectives, rigorously test for biases, and prioritize transparency and explainability in your models.

> **To all stakeholders in the healthcare ecosystem**: foster ongoing dialogue about the ethical implications of AI in medicine.

As these technologies evolve, so must our ethical frameworks. By working together, grounded in the principles of beneficence, non-maleficence, autonomy, and justice, we can create a future where AI enhances rather than diminishes the human elements of healthcare.

The ethical use of LLMs in healthcare is a technical challenge and a societal imperative. Let us rise to this challenge, ensuring that as we push the boundaries of what is possible in medicine, we remain firmly anchored to the ethical principles that have long guided the healing professions. The future of ethical, AI-augmented healthcare is in our hands. Let us shape it wisely.

As we advance into this new era of artificial intelligence in healthcare, from federated learning to large language models, the fundamental principles remain constant: maintain patient privacy, ensure equitable access, preserve clinical judgment, and improve patient outcomes. The technologies we explored in this chapter—from sophisticated machine learning algorithms to ethical frameworks for AI deployment—represent not just tools but stepping stones toward a healthcare system that is more precise, accessible, and humane. The challenge lies not in developing more powerful AI systems but in wielding them wisely.

CHAPTER 3

Multimodal AI

In 1906, Santiago Ramón y Cajal revolutionized our understanding of the brain by integrating multiple ways of seeing. His groundbreaking work combined microscopic observation, detailed drawings, and theoretical insights to reveal how neurons communicate. This multimodal approach to understanding biological systems demonstrated that breakthroughs often come not from a single way of seeing but from combining different perspectives and types of information. More than a century later, we stand at a similar breakthrough moment in healthcare, where artificial intelligence (AI) systems are learning to see and understand patient care through multiple modalities simultaneously.

The rapid and transformative advancements in AI have reshaped various aspects of healthcare. Among these, multimodal AI, a system that integrates multiple data sources such as images, videos, text, and electronic health records (EHRs) to create more comprehensive and accurate models, stands out as a transformative technology. This unique approach to AI is revolutionizing patient care by providing more precise diagnosis, treatment planning, and patient care. Integrating AI in healthcare, particularly in clinical imaging and diagnostics, offers unprecedented opportunities to enhance diagnostic accuracy and streamline clinical workflows.

AI has made significant strides in medical imaging analysis, offering unparalleled accuracy and efficiency in interpreting complex visual data. Deep learning algorithms, particularly convolutional neural networks, have successfully analyzed medical images, such as X-rays, CT scans, and MRIs, to detect abnormalities and assist in diagnosis. For instance, in radiology, AI systems can rapidly analyze chest X-rays to identify lung nodules or signs of pneumonia, reducing the time required for initial screening. In mammography, AI algorithms have shown promise in detecting early signs of breast cancer, improving early diagnosis rates.

A critical advantage of AI in clinical imaging is its ability to process vast amounts of data quickly and consistently. Human radiologists may experience fatigue and variations in performance, but AI algorithms maintain high accuracy and speed, even when dealing with large volumes of images. This capability leads to earlier detection of diseases, more timely interventions, and improved patient outcomes. AI models can detect subtle patterns and anomalies that might be overlooked by human observers, especially in cases of rare conditions or the early stage of disease. This capability is especially valuable in oncology, where early detection improves survival rates.

While AI has made remarkable progress in image analysis, achieving true *seeing*—the ability to understand and interpret visual information in a manner comparable to human cognition—remains currently out of reach. Human cognition requires recognizing patterns and understanding context, causality, and abstract concepts. Medical imaging often involves ambiguous or uncertain cases, such as identifying early signs of a disease or distinguishing between benign and malignant tumors, that require nuanced interpretation.

Developing AI systems that can handle such ambiguity and communicate levels of certainty in their assessments is a crucial area of ongoing research. As AI systems become more complex, ensuring their decisions are interpretable and explainable to healthcare professionals becomes increasingly important. This is critical in high-stakes medical decisions based on visual data analysis.

Holistic Understanding

While AI has shown great promise in analyzing individual data modalities, such as images or text, the true potential of healthcare AI lies in its ability to integrate multiple data sources to create a more holistic understanding of a patient's condition. This potential is where multimodal AI comes into play, combining information from various modalities to generate insights that may be absent when considering each data source in isolation. These systems revolutionize patient care by integrating data from multiple sources, including imaging, sensor data, and EHRs. This integration offers a promising future for healthcare, where patient care is more comprehensive and personalized than ever before.

For example, a multimodal AI system could analyze a patient's CT scans, EHR, and genomic data to provide a more accurate diagnosis and personalized treatment plan for cancer. By considering the patient's medical history, lifestyle factors, and genetic profile alongside the imaging data, the AI system identifies subtle patterns and connections that clinicians may otherwise miss, leading to more precise and effective interventions.

Sidebar: Multimodal Fusion

Multimodal fusion techniques, combining CT imaging data with EHR data, have shown promising results in enhancing the detection of pulmonary embolism. These AI systems provide more accurate and contextual diagnoses by integrating diverse data sources. Clinicians can apply the principles of multimodal fusion to various other diagnostic processes, such as detecting early signs of neurodegenerative diseases by combining brain imaging data with cognitive test results and genetic information. While multimodal fusion offers benefits, we must address the challenges of data standardization, privacy protection, and model complexity before widely adopting these techniques in clinical practice.

In robotic surgery, multimodal AI enhances precision and decision-making by integrating real-time visual data with pre-operative imaging and patient health information. Combining this data leads to more personalized and effective surgical interventions. Multimodal AI also has implications for telemedicine, enabling more accurate remote diagnostics and monitoring. By analyzing visual data from video consultations alongside other health metrics, AI assists healthcare providers in making more informed decisions while offering ongoing guidance to patients.

Beyond Static Images

The application of AI in healthcare is expanding beyond the analysis of static medical images to include video. In surgical settings, AI-powered video provides surgeons with real-time guidance, helping to identify critical structures and complications during procedures. It also helps identify improvements in individual surgeons' surgical techniques, a valuable feedback loop to maintain high levels of surgical competency.

AI-driven video also shows promise in continuous patient monitoring, particularly in intensive care units. It can detect subtle changes in a patient's condition and alert healthcare providers to issues before they become critical.

Visual intelligence is fundamental to human cognition and is crucial in developing advanced AI systems. AI researchers are developing models that mimic the hierarchical structure of the human visual cortex, enabling more sophisticated image analysis and interpretation. Advanced visual AI systems now move beyond simple image recognition to understand context, identify relationships between visual elements, and make complex inferences. This capability is crucial for analyzing pathology slides or interpreting complex radiological images.

Developing AI systems with advanced visual intelligence has implications beyond clinical settings. These technologies can assist in daily living activities for patients with visual impairments or cognitive disorders, enhancing independence and quality of life. In elderly care, AI-powered visual monitoring systems detect falls or unusual behavior patterns, alerting caregivers to emergencies while respecting privacy concerns.

Visual AI can also be used in rehabilitation and physical therapy, providing real-time feedback on patient movements and exercises, ensuring proper form, and tracking progress over time. AI's capability is not just a technological advancement but a strategic investment that improves the quality of patient care and the efficiency of healthcare systems.

Recent advancements in self-supervised learning have demonstrated AI systems' ability to achieve expert-level pathology detection from unannotated chest X-ray images. This approach, which allows AI to learn from vast amounts of unlabeled data, reduces the need for manually annotated datasets in medical imaging AI. A study by Sowrirajan et al. (2021) showed that a self-supervised learning model trained on over 200,000 unlabeled chest X-rays could achieve performance comparable to fully supervised models in detecting conditions such as pneumonia, lung nodules, and cardiomegaly. This breakthrough highlights the potential of AI to leverage the vast amounts of unlabeled medical imaging data available in healthcare systems worldwide.

Bias and Misinformation

> In 1948, the U.S. Public Health Service began the Framingham Heart Study, revolutionizing our understanding of cardiovascular disease. However, its initial focus on a predominantly white, middle-class population led to decades of biased cardiovascular risk assessment for other populations. This historical example reminds us that even well-intentioned medical research can perpetuate biases when based on non-representative populations.

While the potential benefits of multimodal AI are significant, we must ensure its responsible and effective implementation. One of the primary concerns is the explainability and interpretability of AI models. As these systems become more complex and integrate multiple data sources, it becomes increasingly difficult for healthcare professionals to understand how the AI arrived at its conclusions. Developing methods to make AI models more transparent and interpretable is crucial for building trust and ensuring that healthcare providers effectively use these tools in clinical practice.

In addition, it is essential to address the biases that may arise in AI models for clinical imaging. If the training data does not represent the diverse patient population, the AI system may perform poorly or discriminate against certain groups. Ensuring unbiased, diverse, high-quality training data is crucial for developing equitable and reliable AI tools. Regular auditing and testing of AI models across patient populations helps identify and mitigate biases.

Solid ethical principles must guide the development and deployment of healthcare AI. These principles include ensuring patient privacy, obtaining informed consent for data use, and maintaining transparency in how AI systems make decisions. This transparency is not just a requirement but a cornerstone of health-care AI development. It reassures healthcare professionals and patients about the ethical considerations in AI development and is paramount to securing reliable data for AI improving models.

Large, high-quality medical data sets are required to train AI systems properly. Collecting, annotating, and integrating data from various sources is time-consuming, expensive, and subject to privacy and ethical concerns. Furthermore, integrating multimodal AI into clinical workflows requires careful consideration of the impact on healthcare professionals and patients. The negative consequences of automation bias require strict testing and surveillance of the performance of AI systems in clinical workflows. While AI can augment and support human decision-making, it is essential to ensure that healthcare providers retain autonomy and control over the final decisions affecting patient care. Balancing the benefits of AI with the need for human expertise and empathy is a delicate but necessary task.

The theoretical potential of multimodal AI is impressive, but its real value emerges in practical clinical applications. My next *Bedside Consult* examines how computer vision and analytics are already transforming medical imaging, providing concrete examples of how these technologies are being implemented in healthcare settings today. This practical perspective helps bridge the gap between AI's promising capabilities and its actual impact on patient care.

Bedside Consult: How Computer Vision and Analytics is Transforming Medical Imaging

As a physician and a specialist in health information technology, I have witnessed firsthand the transformative power of technology. One such technology that has been making waves in recent years is computer vision. This powerful tool, which allows machines to *see* and interpret visual data, is revolutionizing how we approach healthcare. The following parts aim to shed light on this topic, particularly for large providers, payers, and patients who stand to benefit immensely from these advancements.

Use Cases in Healthcare

Computer vision, a field that falls under the broader umbrella of AI, has been steadily gaining traction in the healthcare sector. It has the capability to drastically improve the way we diagnose diseases, monitor patient health, and even deliver treatments. As a physician, I have seen how this technology enhances diagnostic accuracy, prevents medical errors, and improves patient outcomes.

Automated Image Analysis: Using algorithms to automatically analyze medical images, identify patterns, and detect anomalies. Clinical researchers can train an algorithm to recognize the signs of a stroke in a brain scan. After feeding the algorithm a set of images for review, the analytics generated could include:

- The number of suspected stroke cases properly identified.
- The accuracy of the algorithm.
- The time saved by automating the process.

To apply this, you would need to train a machine-learning model using a large dataset of brain scans, both with and without strokes.

Predictive Analytics: Using historical data to predict future outcomes. By analyzing past mammograms and their associated outcomes, data scientists are building a predictive model to predict the likelihood of breast cancer in future patients. The analytics generated could include:

- The accuracy of the predictions.
- The number of early detections made.
- The impact on patient outcomes.

To apply this, you would need a large dataset of mammograms and associated outcomes and a machine-learning model trained to identify patterns in this data.

Precision Medicine: Analyzing medical images alongside other patient data to develop personalized treatment plans. By analyzing patients' MRI scans and their genetic data, oncologists could create a customized treatment plan for each diagnosed brain tumor. The analytics generated could include:

- The success rate of personalized treatment plans.
- Improvement in patient outcomes.
- Cost-effectiveness of precision medicine.

Tumor Detection and Monitoring: Using analytics to detect tumors in medical images, determine their size and location, and monitor changes over time. Researchers are creating algorithms to detect lung tumors in CT scans and monitor their growth. The analytics generated could include:

- The number of tumors detected.
- The accuracy of the measurements.
- The impact on treatment planning.

Image Segmentation: Separating different structures in medical images, such as organs, tissues, and tumors. Algorithms assist radiologists with segmenting a liver tumor from the surrounding healthy tissue in an MRI scan. Analytics can:

- Improve the accuracy of the segmentation.
- Reduce the time needed to review the scan.
- Enhance surgical planning.

3D Reconstruction: Analyzing multiple 2D images to construct a 3D model of a patient's anatomy. For example, multiple X-ray or CT images could build a 3D model of a patient's spine. The analytics generated could include:

- The accuracy of the 3D models.
- The improvement in surgical planning.
- The impact on patient education.

Comparative Analysis: Comparing a patient's medical images with a database of other images. To aid in the diagnosis, a physician can compare a patient's skin lesion to the images in a skin cancer and benign lesions database. The analytics generated could include:

- The accuracy of the comparative analysis.
- The number of rare or complex conditions identified.
- The impact on patient outcomes.

Quality Control: Using analytics to ensure the quality of medical images. An adequately designed algorithm can identify blurry or improperly aligned X-ray images. The analytics generated could include:

- The number of poor-quality images identified.
- The improvement in image quality.
- The impact on diagnosis accuracy.

Radiomics: Involves extracting many quantitative features from medical images. A radiomics algorithm can identify features from a lung CT scan that predict the response to treatment in lung cancer, assisting the oncologist with treatment planning. The analytics generated for algorithm improvement could include:

- The accuracy of the predictions.
- The number of features extracted.
- The impact on patient prognosis.

Deep Learning: Using machine learning algorithms to analyze medical images and learn from the data. A deep learning model trained to identify signs of diabetic retinopathy in retinal images can assist with diabetic screening. The analytics generated could include:

- The accuracy of the model.
- The number of cases identified.
- The improvement in patient outcomes.

The advent of computer vision in healthcare is a testament to technology's transformative power. As we explore its potential, we can look forward to a future where healthcare is more accurate, efficient, and accessible.

Multimodal artificial intelligence represents a transformative force, combining diverse data sources to enhance clinical decision-making and patient care. From improving diagnostic accuracy through integrated image analysis to enabling more personalized treatment plans, these systems are reshaping how healthcare professionals approach patient care. However, success requires careful attention to bias mitigation, ethical considerations, and preserving human judgment in clinical decision-making. As we continue to develop and implement these technologies, maintaining a balance between innovation and responsible deployment will be crucial for realizing the full potential of multimodal AI while ensuring equitable and effective patient care.

CHAPTER 4

Synergizing AI and Predictive Analytics

In 1855, Florence Nightingale pioneered statistical analysis during the Crimean War to predict and prevent hospital deaths. By meticulously collecting and analyzing mortality data, she demonstrated that poor sanitation was killing more soldiers than battlefield injuries. Her groundbreaking use of statistics and visual diagrams to predict and prevent adverse outcomes established the foundation for data-driven healthcare decision-making. Today, artificial intelligence (AI) extends Nightingale's vision exponentially, processing millions of data points in real time to predict and prevent adverse patient outcomes across entire healthcare systems.

AI has ushered in a new era of healthcare analytics, promising a future of more personalized, efficient, and effective care. Unlike traditional analytics tools, AI-powered predictive analytics can seamlessly integrate into existing healthcare applications and processes. This integration enables healthcare professionals to access real-time insights directly within their workflow, enhancing decision-making and operational efficiency and opening a world of possibilities for improving care delivery.

Predictive analytics is a powerful tool for identifying health risks before they escalate. It is invaluable in critical care settings such as emergency departments, surgical theaters, and intensive care units. By anticipating patient needs and potential complications, predictive analytics allows for more efficient staff allocation and resource optimization, reducing morbidity and ensuring the best possible care for patients.

However, the impact of AI and predictive analytics extends far beyond clinical applications. They are crucial in streamlining operational processes, fostering data-driven decision-making cultures, and improving healthcare delivery systems. The synergy between AI and analytics is reshaping healthcare delivery, promising a future of more personalized, efficient, and effective care.

Recent advancements in AI's analytical power, such as the development of large language models and multimodal AI systems, have further expanded the implementation of AI-driven applications in healthcare. These cutting-edge technologies process and analyze diverse types of medical data, including text, images, and even speech, providing more comprehensive insights for healthcare professionals.

Despite these advancements, challenges remain in integrating AI. While AI excels at processing quantitative data, it must still work on a nuanced understanding of qualitative information, such as patient experiences or subjective symptom descriptions. The complexity of healthcare outcomes, influenced by genetics, lifestyle, and environmental conditions, further complicates AI's ability to predict outcomes accurately without a holistic understanding of these variables.

Moreover, integrating AI necessitates robust measures to ensure data security, patient confidentiality, and informed consent. As AI systems process vast amounts of sensitive health data, it is crucial to implement stringent safeguards to protect patient privacy and maintain public trust in these technologies.

The Internet of Things (IoT) is pivotal in various aspects of healthcare management, from asset tracking to predictive medical equipment maintenance. Hospitals leverage IoT to monitor the status and location of medical devices in real time, ensuring optimal utilization and reducing operational costs. Predictive analytics in IoT help forecast equipment maintenance needs, preventing unexpected breakdowns and ensuring the availability of critical medical equipment when needed most.

It is important to note that the effectiveness of healthcare AI heavily relies on the availability and quality of healthcare data for training models. Similarly, synthetic data—artificially generated data that mimics real patient data without the associated privacy concerns—is becoming increasingly important in healthcare AI development.

Causal Machine Learning

Causal machine learning is emerging as a vital component in advancing care delivery and precision medicine. This sophisticated approach focuses on understanding the causal relationships within medical data, a significant leap beyond traditional predictive analytics. In healthcare, where decision-making and patient outcomes are paramount, causal machine learning offers a more nuanced understanding of why specific treatments work for some patients but not others, providing healthcare professionals with a wealth of new actionable knowledge.

Clinicians can make more informed decisions by identifying the causal factors behind various health conditions and responses to treatments. This method goes beyond predicting patient outcomes based on historical data; it provides insights into diseases' underlying mechanisms and treatments' efficacy. Understanding these causal relationships is crucial in precision medicine, where the objective is to tailor treatments to individual patients. This approach is also beneficial in managing complex, chronic conditions where multiple factors influence the patient's health.

Recent advancements in causal machine learning algorithms have improved their ability to handle high-dimensional data and complex relationships, making them even more suitable for healthcare applications. These improvements allow for a more accurate identification of causal factors in complex diseases and treatment responses.

While causal machine learning helps us understand the *why* behind healthcare outcomes, organizations must also grapple with vast amounts of unused data—often called *dark data*—that hold valuable insights for improving patient care.

Sidebar: Unlocking the Value of Dark Data

Claude Shannon's groundbreaking 1948 paper, "A Mathematical Theory of Communication," revolutionized our understanding of information theory and established the foundation of modern digital communication. Shannon introduced the concept of quantifying information and analyzing it mathematically, paving the way for innovations such as data compression, error correction, and the efficient transmission of information over networks. This seminal work created the bedrock for advancements ranging from the development of the internet to the proliferation of wireless communication technologies that underpin much of our interconnected world today. Just as Shannon expanded our view of how data is used, today's AI tools are transforming how we understand and utilize previously untapped healthcare data.

Dark data refers to information assets organizations collect, process, and store, automatically generated by their operational systems during regular business activities. For example, clerks use point-of-sale systems to collect payment for purchased items. These systems capture data on what items are purchased, which is then used by inventory systems to replenish stock.

Leveraging dark data provides more profound, comprehensive insights into healthcare operations and patient care. For instance, AI can analyze patterns in data like patient interactions, treatment outcomes, or operational efficiency that were previously inaccessible or overlooked.

Implementing AI tools to sift through and make sense of dark data allows healthcare organizations to advance their analytical capabilities. Each step towards a higher level of sophistication in analytics use represents an opportunity for these organizations to derive more business value. It is about converting dark data's hidden patterns and insights into strategic knowledge that informs better patient outcomes, operational efficiencies, and financial performance.

Dark data could range from patient interaction videos and call center recordings to data gathered from IoT devices. These often overlooked data hold valuable insights into patient behavior, treatment efficacy, and staff efficiencies. Applying AI to analyze this data can lead to groundbreaking discoveries in patient care and healthcare management.

Integration of Unstructured Data with Metrics

In 1956, when Allen Newell and Herbert Simon un-
veiled the *Logic Theorist*, a program capable of mimicking human problem-solving, they sparked a revolution
in computational thinking that would eventually evolve
into the field we now call artificial intelligence. Dubbed
the first AI program, the Logic Theorist was designed
to prove mathematical theorems, demonstrating the potential for machines to engage in reasoning processes
traditionally associated with human intelligence. This
breakthrough marked the beginning of a new era where
computers were no longer seen merely as tools for arith-
metic but as systems capable of emulating cognitive
tasks. Their pioneering work in problem-solving laid the
foundation for modern AI's ability to extract meaning
from complex, unstructured information.

Healthcare data is vast and varied, encompassing everything
from patient medical records to real-time monitoring data. Much
of this data is unstructured and complex, making it challenging to
analyze using conventional methods. Recent advancements in natural language processing and computer vision have greatly enhanced
AI's ability to extract meaningful information from unstructured
data sources like medical notes, imaging studies, and patient-generated content. With its advanced algorithms and machine learning capabilities, AI can dissect this data, uncovering patterns and
correlations that would otherwise go unnoticed. By integrating this
rich data with measurable metrics, healthcare professionals better
understand patient health, leading to more accurate diagnoses and
effective treatment plans.

As healthcare organizations increasingly rely on AI to analyze
structured and unstructured data, understanding how these systems

reach their conclusions becomes crucial. This need for transparency leads us to the critical concept of explainable healthcare AI.

Explainable Healthcare AI

In 1976, Edward Shortliffe introduced *MYCIN*, a pioneering expert system designed to assist physicians in diagnosing and recommending treatments for bacterial infections, particularly those involving blood. MYCIN represented a groundbreaking advancement in medical computing and artificial intelligence, as it not only provided diagnostic advice but also explained its reasoning process. Using a rule-based approach, the system leveraged a set of approximately 450 decision-making rules derived from medical expertise. This enabled MYCIN to analyze patient data, recommend potential treatments, and provide a detailed rationale for its conclusions, allowing users to understand the logic behind its decisions.

The need for explainable AI models becomes more pressing as AI is increasingly integrated into healthcare decision-making processes. AI model explanations are crucial for building trust and transparency in AI-assisted healthcare, as they help clinicians understand the reasoning behind AI predictions and recommendations.

Explainable AI models empower clinicians by offering insights into how the model arrived at a particular output, highlighting the key factors and features influencing the decision. These insights are crucial in healthcare, where the stakes are high and the consequences of incorrect or biased decisions are severe. By providing explanations for AI model outputs, clinicians can take an active role in understanding the limitations and biases of the model, thereby making more informed decisions about when to rely on AI recommendations.

One of the key benefits of AI model explanations is their ability to help identify and mitigate systematic biases in AI models. AI models are only as good as the data used for training, and if the training data contains biases or lacks diversity, the model may produce biased or inaccurate outputs. The consequences of such incorrect or biased decisions in healthcare can be life-threatening. By explaining AI model decisions, clinicians can identify instances where the model may rely on inappropriate or irrelevant factors, such as race or gender, and take steps to correct these biases, thereby mitigating some risks.

AI model explanations are essential in image-based medical specialties, such as radiology and pathology, where AI models are increasingly used to assist with diagnosis and treatment planning. In these fields, AI models analyze medical images and identify patterns and features that may be difficult for human clinicians to detect.

AI could greatly enhance medical care by helping doctors make decisions, but doctors may be reluctant to trust AI recommendations that do not explain their reasoning, especially when those recommendations conflict with the doctor's medical judgment.

To address this challenge, researchers are developing new techniques for generating image-based explanations for AI model decisions. These techniques use various methods, such as heat maps and saliency maps, to highlight the regions of the image that the model is focusing on when making its predictions. By providing these visual explanations, clinicians can better understand how the model interprets the image data and identify areas of concern or uncertainty.

However, generating effective and meaningful AI model explanations is not trivial. Explanations must be carefully designed to be accurate and understandable to the intended audience, including clinicians with varying levels of technical expertise. Explanations should also be tailored to the specific clinical context and specialty, considering the patient's medical history, current condition, and treatment options.

Moreover, there are ongoing debates around the trade-offs between model accuracy and interpretability. Some of the most accurate and robust AI models, such as deep learning neural networks, are also the most complex and opaque, making it difficult to generate meaningful explanations for their decisions.

Recent advancements in explainable AI have led to the development of novel techniques such as LIME (Local Interpretable Model-agnostic Explanations) and SHAP (SHapley Additive exPlanations), which aim to provide more intuitive and context-specific explanations for AI model decisions. These techniques are being increasingly applied in healthcare settings to enhance the transparency and interpretability of AI-assisted decision-making processes.

Considerations Moving Forward

Integrating AI and analytics holds immense promise to revolutionize patient care, streamline operations, and drive innovation. As healthcare organizations continue to adopt and refine these technologies, they must consider several key considerations.

First, healthcare organizations should prioritize data quality and standardization. AI and analytics tools are only as effective as the available data. Investing in robust data infrastructure, implementing standardized data collection processes, and regularly cleansing and validating data are crucial steps in ensuring the accuracy and reliability of AI-driven insights.

Second, fostering a culture of collaboration and continuous learning is essential. Implementing AI and analytics requires close cooperation between multi-disciplinary teams, including clinicians, data scientists, IT professionals, and bioethicists. Encouraging open communication, knowledge sharing, and continuous learning helps healthcare organizations stay at the forefront of adopting AI and analytics.

Third, healthcare organizations must remain vigilant in addressing AI's ethical implications. As discussed earlier, data privacy, patient consent, and algorithmic bias are critical ethical considerations that require ongoing attention and proactive management. Establishing clear ethical guidelines, regularly auditing AI systems for fairness, and engaging in open dialogue with patients and the broader healthcare community is essential to ensure the responsible use of AI.

Fourth, synthetic data is becoming increasingly important in AI development. Synthetic data, artificially generated to mimic actual patient data without the associated privacy concerns, offers a promising solution to the data scarcity problem.

Finally, keeping the patient at the center of all AI and analytics initiatives is crucial. While these technologies can transform healthcare delivery, we must always use them to improve patient outcomes and experiences. Engaging patients in the development and deployment of AI tools, providing transparent information about how clinicians use AI in their care, and continuously monitoring the impact of AI on patient satisfaction and outcomes are vital to ensuring that these technologies genuinely benefit patients.

Considering these forward-looking perspectives on AI and analytics, it is important to examine how organizations can practically implement these concepts to achieve measurable value. My next *Bedside Consult* explores strategies for leveraging analytics to optimize value in healthcare settings.

Bedside Consult: Achieve Value Optimization by Effectively Leveraging Analytics

In an era where business consultants refer to data as the *new oil*, effectively harnessing its power is crucial for organizations across various sectors. Embedded analytics and value optimization have emerged as pivotal tools, offering a robust framework for real-time decision-making and efficient resource allocation. These tools are particularly relevant in today's fast-paced, data-driven landscape, where the demand for actionable insights is ever-increasing.

Embedded analytics integrates analytical capabilities within business applications, systems, or processes. Unlike standalone analytics platforms, embedded analytics provides real-time insights directly within the user interface of the tools professionals already use. This seamless integration allows immediate data interpretation and action, reducing the latency often associated with traditional analytics platforms.

Value optimization is not merely about reducing costs; it is a strategic approach focusing on maximizing business value while minimizing wasteful expenditures.

According to Gartner, a 360-degree approach to value optimization involves applying the 80/20 principle, where organizations should concentrate their efforts on the critical 20% of activities that produce 80% of the business value. This approach enables organizations to avoid spending on activities of marginal value, optimizing costs and outcomes. It is a comprehensive strategy that ensures all aspects of the organization are considered for value optimization, leading to maximum efficiency and effectiveness.

For example, in healthcare IT, value optimization can evolve an organization from a traditional *role of keeping the lights on*—maintaining the electronic health record (EHR)—to that of an enterprise process and information architect. This shift allows the organization to focus on business outcomes, such as leveraging data for strategic clinical initiatives rather than just essential IT services.

Organizations can balance cost efficiency and quality by adopting a holistic approach to value optimization, maximizing return on investment (ROI), and enhancing stakeholder satisfaction.

Importance of Embedded Analytics

One of embedded analytics's most compelling advantages is its real-time decision-making capacity. Embedded analytics within the EHR provide clinicians with immediate insights into patient conditions, enabling timely interventions. These quick decisions are crucial in emergency care, treating chronic disease, and managing patients on multiple medications for life-threatening illnesses. Real-time analytics is also invaluable in population health management and public health initiatives, where rapid response to emerging situations, such as outbreaks, is essential.

Embedded analytics improves the user experience by providing actionable insights directly within the applications or platforms with which users are already engaged. Physicians can trend patient results over time and adjust treatment at the point of care when necessary. This trend reduces the need for later follow-up or missed opportunities to properly change care therapies, empowering healthcare professionals and instilling confidence in their decisions.

Data Democratization

Integrating analytics within existing systems facilitates data democratization, empowering all care team members to make data-driven decisions. This data sharing is essential in sectors like healthcare, where multi-disciplinary teams must collaborate for optimal patient outcomes. By making data more accessible and interpretable, embedded analytics builds a culture of informed decision-making across all levels of an organization, fostering a sense of unity and collaboration among team members.

Cost Efficiency and Resource Allocation

Value optimization is intrinsically linked to cost efficiency. Optimizing value could involve strategies to reduce hospital readmissions, which are often costly and indicative of suboptimal care. By leveraging data analytics, healthcare providers can identify patterns and risk factors that lead to readmissions, thereby implementing preventive measures that improve patient outcomes and reduce costs.

Efficient resource allocation manifests as optimized inventory management, where real-time analytics help maintain the right amount of stock to meet demand without incurring additional storage costs or dangerous stockouts. This balance is crucial for maximizing ROI and enhancing patient care.

Role of Predictive Analytics

Predictive analytics is revolutionizing the healthcare industry by enabling providers to anticipate patient needs, allocate resources more effectively, and improve the quality of care. Predictive analytics utilizes data-driven models to identify health risks before they escalate into serious problems. Identifying risk is particularly valuable in emergency care, surgery, and intensive care settings, where quick reactions and timely decision-making impact patient outcomes.

The application of predictive analytics transcends clinical care. It also plays a crucial role in improving operational efficiency by predicting resource requirements, thereby aiding in value optimization. For example, predictive analytics can notify providers when a patient's risk factors indicate a high probability of readmission within 30 days, allowing healthcare systems to allocate resources for outpatient follow-up care more effectively. These notifications improve patient outcomes and have financial implications, as health systems face penalties under programs like Medicare's Hospital Readmissions Reduction Program.

Moreover, predictive analytics is used to personalize treatments based on an individual's medical history or genetic profile. It also helps manage high-risk patients, essential for improving quality and transitioning to value-based care. With machine learning and artificial intelligence, predictive analytics is becoming an increasingly sophisticated tool that approximates the probability of various outcomes based on historical data. These predictions allow clinicians, financial analysts, and administrative personnel to make forward-thinking decisions.

Use Case: Sepsis

The management and outcomes of sepsis patients are of paramount importance. The Centers for Disease Control and Prevention (CDC) recently updated its core elements for hospital sepsis programs, which include hospital leadership commitment, accountability, multi-professional expertise, action, tracking, reporting, and education. Embedded analytics within EHR systems is pivotal in enhancing these core elements.

For instance, a hospital in Massachusetts implemented embedded analytics in its EHR system to align with the CDC's core elements for sepsis care. The analytics tool flagged high-risk patients for sepsis in real time, aiding in recognizing sepsis as emphasized by the CDC. This real-time tracking and reporting facilitated the implementation of evidence-based management strategies, aligning with the *action* and *tracking* core elements.

The embedded analytics also supported patients' recovery after sepsis by monitoring various health parameters and alerting healthcare providers for timely interventions. This improved patient outcomes and optimized value in terms of reduced hospital mortality, length of stay, and healthcare costs, consistent with the benefits observed in hospital quality improvement programs focused on sepsis.

By integrating embedded analytics into EHR systems, hospitals can enhance their sepsis care programs, aligning them with the CDC's guidelines and making them more effective in improving patient outcomes and optimizing healthcare costs.

Embedded analytics offers the advantage of real-time decision-making, enhanced user experience, and data democratization. At the same time, value optimization maximizes ROI through cost efficiency, resource allocation, and quality improvement. The synergy between these two concepts fosters a data-driven culture, enabling predictive analytics that further enhances performance and outcomes.

Embedded analytics and value optimization are not merely trends but essential strategies for organizations aiming to thrive in a data-driven landscape. Future research and development should leverage these tools for more personalized, efficient, and ethical solutions across all sectors.

Integrating artificial intelligence and predictive analytics in healthcare represents a transformative opportunity to enhance patient care, improve operational efficiency, and drive innovation. By carefully considering the technical, ethical, and practical aspects of implementation while maintaining a focus on explainability and value optimization, healthcare organizations can harness these powerful tools to create a more effective and patient-centered healthcare system. As we look to the future, the synergy between human expertise and AI will continue to evolve, offering new possibilities for improving healthcare delivery and outcomes. The key to success lies in maintaining a balanced approach that embraces technological advancement while preserving the essential human elements of healthcare delivery.

CHAPTER 5

AI in Healthcare Delivery

In 1954, Dr. Homer Warner began his work using computers for decision support in cardiology at Intermountain's LDS Hospital in Salt Lake City. The program assisted clinicians by using medical logic to evaluate patient data. It could generate alerts, reminders, and messages, and provide suggestions for interventions. Seven decades later, we are at a similar inflection point, where artificial intelligence (AI) now detects patterns across vast arrays of medical data, from complex imaging studies to intricate genomic sequences, transforming our ability to understand and treat disease.

AI's capacity to analyze complex medical data and identify patterns enables it to diagnose diseases. Recent advancements have further improved AI's diagnostic capabilities, with some models achieving performance levels comparable to or exceeding human experts.

Machine learning and natural language processing (NLP) are at the forefront of enhancing clinical judgment. These AI components enable healthcare systems to process vast datasets, learning and adapting from each interaction. With their ability to continually learn from data rather than follow predefined rules, machine learning algorithms rapidly evolve to become more accurate. This adaptability differs from practice guidelines that are relatively fixed and not representative of each patient's uniqueness.

AI's most notable impact is in medical imaging. Advanced AI algorithms can interpret various medical images, from chest radiographs detecting pneumonia to histopathology images for cancer diagnosis. There are also emerging AI applications in interventional radiology, assisting in real-time image guidance during minimally invasive procedures. These AI systems can accurately identify abnormalities, often at par or even superior to human experts.

AI's effectiveness is more pronounced in cases where clinical diagnoses are more objective or numerically defined, such as a significant rise in creatinine levels indicating acute kidney injury. However, clinical diagnosis often involves interpreting a mix of imprecise, non-numerical data and patient symptoms, where objective pathognomonic tests may not exist. Many medical conditions require more definitive confirmatory tests, making the final diagnosis often a matter of clinical consensus rather than objective confirmation. AI's utility is limited in such scenarios, as it is more suited to conditions with clear, numerical diagnostic criteria.

Clinical diagnosis is an art that involves more than just interpreting data; it requires fundamental clinical skills such as history taking and physical examination. For instance, a clinician's assessment of jugular venous pressure or detection of suprapubic tenderness influences a diagnosis. These skills provide context and nuances that are often beyond the current scope of AI.

For many medical conditions, such as cellulitis, pneumonia, or heart failure, reaching a conclusive diagnosis relies heavily on the clinician's judgment rather than a definitive test. This subjective nature of diagnosis makes it challenging to assess the accuracy of

AI in these scenarios. Currently, AI cannot replicate these nuanced assessments, critical in forming an accurate clinical picture.

To address this challenge, researchers are developing AI systems integrating multiple data sources, including imaging, lab results, and clinical notes, to provide a more comprehensive diagnostic assessment. These systems aim to mimic the holistic approach of experienced clinicians, who consider various factors in their diagnostic process.

Recent research has focused on developing AI systems that handle uncertainty and provide probabilistic diagnoses, an approach Dr. Larry Weed pioneered with his *Problem Knowledge Coupler* more than 40 years ago. These systems offer a range of potential diagnoses with associated confidence levels, mirroring the thought process of experienced clinicians and providing a more nuanced approach to AI-assisted diagnosis and therapeutic planning.

The ongoing development and integration of AI models into clinical workflows can enhance the quality of care and patient outcomes. However, it is vital to address biases in AI models, ensure the accuracy of predictions, and maintain a collaborative approach between AI tools and clinicians. This collaborative approach ensures that AI is not a replacement for clinical judgment but a powerful tool that augments and enhances it.

⁂

Current research focuses on developing AI systems that continuously learn and adapt in clinical settings, incorporating new data and feedback from clinicians to improve their performance over time. There is also growing interest in using AI to predict the onset of advanced disease before clinical signs become apparent, allowing for earlier intervention and improved outcomes.

AI's role in medical note dictation is a significant leap in healthcare documentation. Integrating more sophisticated NLP and computer vision techniques has transformed how clinicians interact with electronic health records (EHRs). Leveraging NLP, AI can accurately transcribe, summarize, and highlight key points from patient-doctor conversations, making the documentation process more efficient and accurate.

Advanced NLP models also understand context and nuance in clinical notes, extract relevant information, and turn unstructured data into actionable insights. These systems identify crucial clinical information, red flags, and follow-up items, helping clinicians focus on the most critical aspects of patient care while providing a more accurate and complete medical record. This capability saves time and reduces the risk of overlooking critical information in patient records. However, these systems cannot fully replicate seasoned clinicians' intuition and experience.

Patient Experience, Customer Engagement, and Clinical Operations

In 1962, Dr. Morris Collen, a visionary in medical informatics, introduced the first automated medical history system at Kaiser Permanente. This groundbreaking innovation allowed patients to input their symptoms and medical history directly into a computer before meeting with their physician. The system then organized the information to aid clinicians in diagnosing and treating patients more efficiently. At a time when computers were still relatively novel in healthcare, this initiative demonstrated a forward-thinking approach to integrating technology into medical practice to improve efficiency and patient care. Dr. Collen's work marked one of the earliest attempts to streamline medical documentation. It presaged today's AI-powered documentation systems that transcribe, analyze, and contextualize entire patient encounters in real time.

AI enhances the patient experience by automating and optimizing administrative functions, facilitating more efficient patient-provider interactions. This enhancement extends to personalized patient outreach and education, ensuring patients receive tailored information and customized care pathways, thereby improving the overall quality of care.

New telemedicine platforms integrated with AI algorithms now analyze data obtained through remote patient monitoring and suggest medication adjustments to clinicians. These systems identify trends requiring human intervention, leading to more proactive and precise patient care.

Conversational AI led to more sophisticated chatbots and virtual assistants capable of providing personalized health information and support. These AI-powered tools answer patient queries, provide medication reminders, and even offer mental health support, improving patient engagement and adherence to treatment plans.

AI is also revolutionizing patient interactions with healthcare systems and insurers. AI-driven apps provide personalized health tips, while chatbots assist in appointment scheduling, making healthcare more accessible. These tools offer tailored advice and reminders for medication adherence.

AI-powered health apps have introduced more sophisticated features like emotion recognition and personalized mental health support. These advancements allow for more nuanced and empathetic digital interactions.

AI impacts clinical operations by assisting in managing patient flow, reducing wait times, and improving staff allocation. Recent advancements in AI-driven operational optimization have led to improvements in hospital efficiency. For example, AI-powered predictive models forecast patient admission rates, helping hospitals manage staffing and resource allocation more effectively. These forecasts reduce overcrowding in emergency departments and improve overall patient care quality and satisfaction. AI is also used for capacity management, optimizing operating room workflows, and enhancing supply chain efficiency.

AI provides insights into healthcare data, clarifying patient demographics, disease trends, and treatment outcomes. This information is crucial for healthcare providers and policymakers to make informed decisions on resource planning, budgeting, and disease management programming.

For insurers and patients, AI simplifies the complex processes of insurance verification, claims processing, and coverage determination. Vendors are developing new AI-powered systems to predict insurance claim outcomes and suggest optimal coding practices, reducing claim denials and improving reimbursement rates. These systems also assist patients in understanding their insurance benefits and out-of-pocket costs, promoting transparency and informed decision-making by patients.

While AI demonstrates remarkable capabilities in analyzing healthcare data and supporting clinical decisions, its effectiveness ultimately depends on the quality of its training data. The critical dependency between AI performance and data quality raises important considerations about the accuracy and reliability of EHRs, which serve as the primary data source for many clinical AI applications.

Sidebar: Accuracy of EHR Data

Using AI in healthcare necessitates a rigorous and accurate collection of training data, as the efficacy of AI tools depends heavily on the precision of the data they analyze. This precision is vital for rare or complex cases and common conditions where diagnostic errors have profound implications. The consequences of unreliable EHR data are far-reaching. AI models trained on this data perpetuate and even exacerbate inaccuracies, leading to diagnostic and therapeutic errors.

EHRs contain inaccuracies due to practices like copying and pasting, leading to bloated EHRs often containing replicated inaccurate clinical notes. Thus, the effectiveness of AI depends as much on the integrity of the data it analyzes as on the sophistication and training of its algorithms.

Recent advancements in AI technology have led to developing systems that identify and account for data quality issues. These systems use advanced machine learning techniques to detect inconsistencies or anomalies in EHR data, adjusting their diagnostic confidence accordingly and flagging data quality concerns for human review. These systems identify data quality issues and provide clinicians with transparency about the certainty of their predictions.

Additional data improvement initiatives focus on improving the quality of EHR data at the point of care. Advanced NLP tools are being developed to assist clinicians in real time, suggesting corrections and standardizations as they input data into EHR systems. This approach aims to improve data quality at the source, enhancing the reliability of AI-generated insights.

Do No Harm

While AI promises to enhance patient care, accurately judging its effectiveness remains complex. The inherent ambiguities in clinical diagnosis and treatments, as well as the challenges of ensuring data accuracy, highlight the need for careful evaluation before integrating AI in healthcare. Ongoing research focuses on developing more robust evaluation methodologies and creating AI systems that operate effectively in the face of clinical ambiguity and data quality issues.

Healthcare AI raises essential ethical considerations, such as how AI recommendations should be integrated into clinical decision-making and how these systems account for the nuances of individual patient care. Current discussions in the field are centered around developing ethical guidelines for AI, ensuring transparency in AI decision-making processes, and maintaining patient privacy and data security. There is also ongoing work to improve the interpretability of AI models, making their decision-making processes more understandable to healthcare providers and patients.

When Dr. Larry Weed introduced *SOAP* notes in 1964, he sought to standardize medical documentation to improve information sharing among healthcare providers. Today, as we grapple with AI implementation and data standardization, we face similar fundamental challenges in effectively structuring and sharing clinical information. The historical parallel between healthcare standardization efforts and other industries proves particularly instructive. My next *Bedside Consult* explores how the 19th-century challenge of railroad gauge standardization mirrors our current struggle with healthcare data interoperability. This challenge becomes increasingly critical as AI systems require consistent, standardized data to function effectively.

Bedside Consult: Railroads, Weed, and EHRs

As independent companies built railroad lines in the 19th century, each chose a different gauge—the distance between the inner rails—for their track. As the railway industry first grew out of the need to transport mined materials, most early railroad companies chose a gauge that approximated the distance between the wheels of a horse-drawn cart. Similarly, as EHR companies built their software, they chose proprietary standards for data elements, database architecture, and exchange of patient information.

The standard gauge—also known as the Stephenson gauge (named after George Stephenson, inventor of the first steam-powered railroad locomotive), international gauge, or normal gauge—makes up more than 60% of all railroad tracks worldwide. In the

United States, Canada, and Britain, the distance between the rails is 4 feet 8½ inches, and in the rest of the world, 1,435 mm, with the latter representing approximately a ½ mm variance and acceptable track tolerance.

Although track gauge varied widely throughout the 19th century, sparking many *gauge wars*, an 1845 Royal Commission of the United Kingdom, Great Britain, and Ireland set the standard gauge at 4 feet 8½ inches rather than the competing 7-foot gauge proposed by the Great Western Railway.

Even though the wider gauge used by the Great Western Railway offered greater passenger comfort, larger carrying loads, and more efficient transport of passengers and goods, the Royal Commission rejected the gauge simply because most of the track in the UK conformed to the four ft. 8½ inch standard.

Today, our EHR systems, designed on a proprietary framework to primarily capture clinical documentation to optimize payment and secondarily record patient care, need to improve exchanging personal health information and presenting patient data to drive high-quality, efficient patient care. Like the railroad gauge, EHR standards evolved from commercial interests unrelated to the best possible technology or desired public outcomes.

Learning from Weed

The effort to design frameworks to document care in a systematic way to help deliver better clinical outcomes began in 1964 when Dr. Larry Weed, in the *Irish Journal of Medical Science,* described *SOAP notes*, a structure for documenting medical care organized around four key areas:

Subjective: Information obtained directly from the patient, including the patient's chief complaint or reason for the visit.

Objective: Factual information about the patient, including vital signs, data obtained from physical exam, and lab values.

Assessment: A medical diagnosis for the patient visit (or differential diagnosis if unsure of the final diagnosis) with a factual explanation of the decision-making.

Plan: Description of the treatment steps addressing each diagnosis/problem independently.

At that time, clinicians used highly personalized formats for documenting patient care, which proved unwieldy and of dubious value for sharing patient information with other providers. With SOAP notes, Dr. Weed established an exchangeable standard for documenting care that allowed easier sharing of patient data and clinical reasoning among clinicians.

Four years later, Dr. Weed wrote a sentinel article in *The New England Journal of Medicine* titled "Medical records that guide and teach." In that article, Dr. Weed laid out his reasoning for standardizing the organization of a patient's medical record:

> "... it will be necessary to develop a more organized approach to the medical record, a more rational acceptance and use of paramedical personnel, and a more positive attitude about the computer in medicine."

> "Among physicians, there has been uncritical adherence to the first phase of medical action, which is the collection of data, upon which complete formulation and management of all the patient's problems depends."

In the early 1970s, Dr. Weed further developed his structured documentation approach and described the *problem-oriented medical record (POMR)*. Based on his SOAP note method, this approach organized the medical record around patient problems with an underlying structure. Over many years of evangelizing by Dr. Weed and others, the POMR and its underlying SOAP structure became the *de facto standard* for documenting patient care. Nevertheless, this *standard* is not universally applied by all organizations and clinicians.

The Wrong Standard

The POMR and SOAP notes were based on unstructured data (e.g., physician notes), so health information technology companies built their EHR systems to accommodate this unstructured data approach to clinical documentation rather than develop a new system of documentation that would have leveraged information technology capabilities. Although Dr. Weed advocated this unstructured method for paper-based clinical documentation, he envisioned a time when computers would eliminate the need for unstructured data. In his 1968 article referenced above, he predicted:

> "It can readily be seen that all narrative data presently in the medical record can be structured, and in the future, all narrative data may be entered through a series of displays, guaranteeing a thoroughness, retrievability, efficiency, and economy important to the scientific analysis of a type of datum that has hitherto been handled in a very unrigorous manner."

Today, organizations and clinicians cling to the importance of unstructured records and refuse to consider a new approach to digital clinical documentation. Data scientists espouse the value of NLP to release the value of the information contained within the unstructured medical record data.

Perhaps it is time to heed the advice of Dr. Weed and construct a new approach to electronic documentation of the patient record that focuses on promoting the best patient care while reducing the burden of electronic documentation on physicians, nurses, and all other clinical providers. In addition, the clinical data requires a format that is genuinely interchangeable in a clinically meaningful way that directly drives patient care rather than remain hidden in a hard-to-utilize, verbose format that satisfies the technical criteria of clinical information exchange. Clinical care does not suffer from a paucity of patient information. The opposite is true as clinicians need help identifying useful information among the tsunami of insignificant data.

Reboot the EHR

EHRs currently contain more information than clinicians have time to either review or synthesize. Our EHRs mimic clinical care workflow in a paper-based, clinical documentation world rather than one that leverages the best information systems. EHRs burden clinicians with documentation tasks that have little or no impact on clinical outcomes. In some instances, the documentation burden lowers the effectiveness of the clinical encounter, thereby reducing the quality of patient care.

EHRs require a reboot; the clinical documentation workflow should be redesigned to leverage the information flowing from the EHR and other integrated systems. Engaging user experiences that use existing, familiar technologies that are part of our everyday experience must be employed to present meaningful, digestible, and actionable patient data and collect additional patient information for future use. The clinical workflow of next-generation EHR systems will also use medical knowledge from guidelines and algorithms to request useful documentation from the clinician and present meaningful information to the clinician.

As the number of sources of patient data expands from the clinical setting to the personal realm of smart devices and sensors, clinicians require a documentation system that organizes all this data into a useful package that can effectively help direct patient care. Burdening clinicians with documentation tasks driven by an outdated paper-based approach to medical records seems foolish and wasteful. We must discard the *standard gauge and* move on to a *better gauge* for clinical documentation that puts patient care first while lessening the unproductive documentation burden currently assigned to clinicians. In addition, the presentation of patient data should be synthesized and formatted to allow for maximum utility by the clinician in the delivery of patient care.

The evolution of healthcare technology, from the first medical computer in 1954 to today's sophisticated artificial intelligence systems, reflects remarkable progress. The future success of healthcare AI depends not just on algorithmic sophistication but on our ability to reimagine how we collect, standardize, and utilize clinical information. This transformation requires balancing technical innovation with practical clinical needs, ensuring data quality while reducing documentation burden, and maintaining the essential human elements of healthcare delivery. As healthcare delivery becomes increasingly digital and data-driven, we must resist the temptation to layer AI atop existing workflows and documentation practices.

Just as the standardization of railroad gauges eventually enabled seamless continental travel, the thoughtful integration of artificial intelligence—built on standardized, high-quality clinical data—can help realize the promise of more efficient, effective, and accessible healthcare delivery. However, this can only occur if we focus on redesigning our approach to clinical documentation and data collection to serve patient care rather than perpetuating practices that originated in a paper-based world.

Chapter 6
Augmenting Human Expertise

In 1816, French physician René Laennec revolutionized medical diagnostics with his invention of the *stethoscope*, a simple tool crafted from a rolled-up piece of paper. This innovation allowed doctors to hear internal sounds of the heart and lungs more clearly, enhancing diagnostic accuracy while respecting patient modesty—an issue when placing an ear directly on a patient's chest. The stethoscope became the first tool to augment physicians' senses without replacing their clinical expertise, ushering in a new era of technological integration in medicine. Today, we are at a similar turning point with artificial intelligence (AI) in healthcare. AI tools, like Dr. Laennec's invention, extend clinicians' abilities, offering unprecedented insights into diagnostics, patient monitoring, and treatment planning. By complementing—not replacing—medical expertise, AI represents the next evolution in leveraging technology to enhance patient care.

AI's strength lies in its ability to rapidly analyze vast amounts of data. Modern natural language processing algorithms can sift through unstructured text, identifying patterns and extracting crucial medical information that takes a human practitioner considerably longer to process. This capability allows for a more comprehensive review of a patient's medical history, uncovering overlooked details or connections that could be vital for diagnosis and treatment.

Advancements in large language models enhance AI's capacity to understand and generate human-like text. These models now engage in more natural, context-aware conversations, improving the quality of automated history-taking systems. For instance, AI-powered chatbots can conduct initial patient interviews, asking relevant follow-up questions based on the patient's responses and medical history.

AI's role in collecting patient history complements rather than replaces clinicians' efforts. Documenting a patient's history is not merely about collecting data; it is an intricate dance of communication that involves interpreting nonverbal cues and building a foundation of trust to obtain the most valuable information. These nuanced aspects of human interaction remain beyond AI's current capabilities.

The future use of AI to obtain a patient history lies in a hybrid approach, where AI systems work alongside healthcare providers. For example, AI could conduct initial interviews and data gathering, providing clinicians with a comprehensive summary before they meet the patient. This approach allows healthcare providers to focus on the more nuanced aspects of patient interaction, using the AI-gathered information as a springboard for deeper, more targeted discussions.

Advancements in multimodal AI systems can simultaneously process and analyze various data types, such as text, speech, and images, allowing for a more holistic patient history. These systems can interpret facial expressions, tone of voice, and other nonverbal cues, bringing AI closer to replicating human-like interaction.

AI and Physical Examination Findings

When physician and composer Dr. Leopold Auenbrugger introduced percussion as a diagnostic technique in 1761, he demonstrated how systematic physical examination could reveal internal conditions. In his text *Inventum Novum*, he explained percussing the chest. One passage reads, "For in truth, through these techniques, a sound is perceived either higher or lower or more or less clear or even almost stifled." In retrospect, it is unsurprising that a musician was the first to tap on the chest and use percussion in physical diagnosis.

While AI has made significant strides in assisting with care delivery, its usefulness continues to depend on humans. Physical examinations conducted by skilled healthcare providers remain a cornerstone of patient assessment. These examinations involve complex interpretations and evaluations that AI cannot fully replicate. The nuanced visual and auditory observations made during a physical exam are critical inputs that inform decision-making. Clinicians base these observations on years of experience and a deep understanding of human behavior, making it difficult for AI to replicate.

Leveraging computer vision and deep learning has remarkable pattern recognition and image analysis capabilities, which help AI systems alert clinicians to areas that require attention, supplementing their clinical skills and improving the quality and consistency of exams.

In addition, the use of AI in medical education is training the next generation of healthcare providers. AI-powered simulation systems provide medical students with virtual patients to interview and examine, offering immediate feedback and helping them hone their clinical skills.

While these technological advances enhance clinical capabilities, they highlight a fundamental aspect of healthcare that technology alone cannot replicate—the human capacity for empathy. As we incorporate increasingly sophisticated AI tools into clinical practice, understanding the unique value of human connection becomes even more important.

Sidebar: The Empathy Factor

As healthcare embraces AI, it becomes increasingly clear that human interaction remains irreplaceable. Empathy, an inherent aspect of in-person communication, is vital to deliver quality patient care. It involves understanding patients' emotional and psychological needs, building trust, and providing comfort. Clinicians' ability to connect with patients on a human level, understand their fears and concerns, and offer reassurance is something that AI cannot fully replicate with current technology.

AI tools cannot genuinely understand and respond to human emotions with the depth and nuance of a human caregiver. However, some AI systems recognize emotional cues in speech and text, alerting healthcare providers to patients experiencing anxiety or distress. For instance, AI systems can interpret changes in a patient's tone of voice during a phone call or identify keywords in a patient's text. Even if healthcare AI cannot directly provide empathy, these tools help clinicians determine when patients need additional emotional support.

AI-powered virtual assistants act as companions for patients, augmenting the support offered by families and caregivers. For instance, chatbots designed for mental health can engage in supportive conversations and guide patients through basic cognitive behavioral therapy exercises.

Bridging Distances: Remote Patient Management

In 1905, Dutch physiologist Dr. Willem Einthoven made history by transmitting the first electrocardiogram from a hospital to his laboratory 1.5 kilometers away using telephone cables. This groundbreaking innovation demonstrated the potential of technology to overcome physical barriers, laying the foundation for remote patient monitoring. Einthoven's invention of the electrocardiograph, for which he won the Nobel Prize in 1924, allowed clinicians to study heart activity with unprecedented precision. Today, AI-enabled remote care systems build on Einthoven's pioneering work, facilitating real-time monitoring, diagnosis, and treatment across vast distances, improving access to patient care.

Healthcare AI's advancements in remote patient management greatly benefit patients with chronic conditions who are located large distances away from medical facilities. For example, these systems can educate diabetics on how best to manage their glucose levels and guide them in the use of automated insulin delivery systems.

AI-powered chatbots provide personalized responses to patient queries, offering real-time support and guidance. These chatbots use patients' health data to provide contextual advice based on individual health metrics and treatment plans.

Moreover, AI algorithms can analyze patient electronic health records to predict complications or health issues before they become severe. In diabetes management, AI can analyze blood glucose readings, insulin doses, and lifestyle factors to predict hypoglycemic events, allowing for preemptive interventions.

The shift towards AI-enabled remote patient care helps address the shortages of primary care physicians. By allowing patients to learn and manage their conditions more independently, these systems reduce the need for frequent in-person visits, thus conserving valuable time for healthcare providers to address the needs of other patients.

Healthcare AI facilitates telemedicine by triaging patients for appointments and prioritizing those needing immediate attention. AI tools also enhance the quality of telemedicine visits by providing real-time language translation services.

AI at Your Fingertips

In 1972, Hewlett-Packard released the *HP-35*, the first handheld scientific calculator, revolutionizing how individuals performed complex calculations. Compact yet powerful, the HP-35 replaced the cumbersome slide rule, democratizing access to advanced computational tools for engineers, scientists, and students. This groundbreaking innovation marked a paradigm shift, enabling unprecedented portability and efficiency in number crunching and problem-solving. Similarly, today's *mobile health (mHealth)* applications bring advanced health management tools directly to patients. These applications empower users to monitor vital signs, track fitness goals, and manage chronic conditions, fundamentally transforming healthcare by providing personalized, real-time support.

m-Health applications are important in disease management and lifestyle modification. These applications offer unprecedented benefits, empowering patients with real-time health monitoring, diet tracking, and medication adherence tools.

The advantage of m-Health applications lies in their accessibility and user-friendly interfaces. They bring health management assistance to patients when it is needed. This access is equally valuable for individuals living in remote, underserved areas, or those near healthcare facilities.

With machine learning algorithms, m-Health applications can analyze user data to provide personalized diet, exercise, and medication management recommendations. Some applications predict blood glucose levels based on historical data on eating habits, helping diabetics make better-informed insulin dosing decisions. The integration of AI-powered image recognition in m-Health applications gives patients the ability to use a photo of their meal to obtain its nutritional content and potential impact on their blood glucose levels.

For patients to maximize the benefits of m-Health, the applications should be intuitive and provide evidence-based information. They require flexibility to satisfy users' diverse needs, considering factors like age, cultural background, and technological literacy. Increased data sharing between patients and healthcare providers will further increase their versatility.

Healthcare AI, leveraging advanced natural language processing capabilities, transforms how healthcare professionals communicate clinical information with patients. AI tools simplify complex medical terminologies and generate patient-friendly explanations of diagnoses, treatment plans, and medication instructions tailored to individual needs. This capability enhances patient engagement and education, leading to better healthcare outcomes through improved understanding and adherence to treatment plans.

In addition to providing diagnostic and treatment advice to patients, AI systems can provide clinicians with real-time guidance during medical procedures. For instance, AI-powered imaging systems assist surgeons by highlighting critical structures or suggesting optimal approaches during minimally invasive surgeries. These systems act as an additional set of eyes, improving patient outcomes and reducing complications. They also serve as a data source that leads to improved surgical techniques. Wherever deployed, healthcare must seamlessly integrate into clinical workflows and not disrupt patient care.

The use of AI in care delivery marks an exciting frontier that fundamentally enhances, rather than replaces, human clinical expertise. Yet the successful implementation of these technologies requires healthcare organizations to manage numerous challenges. In my next *Bedside Consult*, I explore how organizations can effectively deploy digital health technologies while ensuring appropriate governance, workflow integration, and protection of patient privacy.

Bedside Consult: Transformative Digital Health Tech

The emergence of wearable digital health technologies (DHTs) can revolutionize healthcare by providing personalized, data-driven insights into patients' health and well-being. As these technologies progress from experimental applications to routine use in clinical care, healthcare stakeholders must address several critical challenges to realize their full potential.

Data ownership and patient privacy remain primary concerns regarding the use of DHTs. Patients require free access to their data and maintain control over its use. They are the sole owners of their health data and must provide informed consent to share it for medical research or commercial product development.

A *digital health counselor*, akin to a genetics counselor, may be needed to assist patients and clinicians with integrating technology, including facilitating access, teaching digital literacy skills, and interpreting clinically relevant data. Additionally, healthcare organizations should implement robust security measures to protect patient information from unauthorized access and breaches, ensuring the utmost respect for patient privacy.

Ensure Interoperability

Effective use of DHTs demands full interoperability. The need for widely adopted standards, such as those developed by the Institute of Electrical and Electronics Engineers, can lead to removing data-sharing barriers and advancing the ability of DHTs to improve patient care. We must reject proprietary data formats that hinder interoperability. The Food and Drug Administration (FDA) provides guidelines for determining which *mobile medical applications* qualify as medical devices and require regulatory oversight, ensuring that these devices are safe, effective, and interoperable.

However, it is not a task for a single entity. Collaborative efforts among healthcare providers, technology companies, and regulatory bodies are necessary to establish and enforce these standards, making everyone feel included in this transformative process. The Office of the National Coordinator for Healthcare Information Technology is responsible for fostering interoperability, so it is best equipped to bring together relevant stakeholders to establish standards.

Further research is needed to fully understand the impact of DHTs on patient care and outcomes. Studies should focus on identifying the specific data points and devices that offer the most significant benefits in various clinical contexts. By leveraging the power of analytics and AI, researchers can uncover best practices for integrating DHTs into clinical workflows, optimizing their value while minimizing disruptions.

Prioritize Clinical Workflow

As DHTs generate vast amounts of data, physicians need to be able to incorporate this information into their clinical workflow effectively. Organizations must ensure that the data presented to physicians is valuable and actionable rather than requiring them to discern its relevance in patient care. AI can address this issue by identifying the most useful data points and devices and determining the most effective ways to utilize them within acceptable clinical workflows. AI algorithms can analyze patterns and correlations within the data, providing physicians with actionable insights to support their decision-making process. However, ongoing investigation is required to identify the most effective way for DHTs to present data to healthcare professionals and patients.

Benefits and Risks

A study in *The New England Journal of Medicine*, "Key issues as wearable digital health technologies enter clinical care" (Ginsburg, 2024) showed that patients with diabetes who use an open-source, community-built smartphone app that captures glucose and insulin pump data from commercial devices improves their insulin control by adjusting their insulin levels more frequently. This study demonstrates the potential for DHTs to empower patients and improve health outcomes.

While DHTs hold great promise for personalizing patient care, it is essential to recognize the risks and challenges associated with their implementation. False alarms from wearable DHTs, such as smartwatches that monitor heart rhythm, may lead to unnecessary medical evaluations and increased healthcare utilization. AI methods have shown promise in reducing false alarms, especially when using large, high-quality data sets for training. Healthcare organizations and DHT companies must prioritize advancing medical research and improving care quality, safety, and access while mitigating risk.

Reimbursement and return on investment for healthcare systems are significant factors in the widespread adoption of DHTs. Evidence of clinical effectiveness and cost savings is needed to justify the investment in these technologies. There is now a set of Current Procedural Terminology (CPT) codes for remote patient monitoring with wearables, which cover FDA-cleared or FDA-approved devices, their setup and patient education, remote monitoring, data reading, and patient consultations. However, devices and procedures that do not meet existing CPT definitions still present severe challenges in securing reimbursement.

Stakeholder Collaboration

As the adoption of DHTs continues to grow, ongoing collaboration among healthcare providers, technology developers, policymakers, and patient advocates is essential. By working together to address the complex challenges surrounding DHT integration, including informed consent, data security, patient control, interoperability, and clinical workflow integration, we can create a future in which these technologies seamlessly complement traditional medical practices.

Earlier interventions, more proactive disease management, and a greater emphasis on preventive measures made possible by DHTs can reduce the burden of chronic conditions, prevent costly hospitalizations, and optimize resource allocation. By harnessing the power of DHTs, we can empower patients and providers alike to make informed, data-driven decisions that lead to better health outcomes for all while advancing the vision of precision medicine.

The journey from Laennec's simple stethoscope to today's AI-powered healthcare systems reflects a consistent truth in medicine—technology works best when it amplifies rather than replaces human capabilities. As we have explored throughout this chapter, AI serves as a powerful amplifier of clinical expertise—augmenting our ability to gather patient histories, conduct physical examinations, manage remote care, and deliver mobile health solutions. However, successful integration of these technologies requires careful attention to both technical and human factors:

- Maintaining empathetic patient care.
- Ensuring seamless workflow integration.
- Protecting privacy.
- Establishing appropriate governance frameworks.

The experiences shared in my *Bedside Consult* underscore a crucial point. While AI and DHTs offer transformative change, their success depends on thoughtful implementation that prioritizes patient needs and clinical workflows. As healthcare continues its digital transformation, organizations must strike a delicate balance—leveraging AI's analytical power while preserving the irreplaceable human elements of care. The future of healthcare lies not in choosing between human expertise and artificial intelligence but in creating synergistic partnerships where each complements the other's strengths in providing high-quality patient care.

CHAPTER 7

Virtual Assistants

In 1952, engineers Stephen Balashek, R. Biddulph, and K. H. Davis at Bell Labs developed *Audrey* (short for Automatic Digit Recognizer), a groundbreaking system capable of recognizing spoken digits with remarkable accuracy. Audrey could identify the numbers 0 through 9 with 90% precision, a significant achievement in an era when computers were still in their infancy. This early speech recognition system was designed to respond to the voice of a single speaker and required extensive training. Still, its development represented a pivotal step in enabling machines to understand and process human speech, laying the foundation for modern speech technology.

Virtual assistants (VAs) offer a unique blend of artificial intelligence (AI) and user interface to support various aspects of healthcare delivery. Unlike broader AI applications discussed in previous chapters, VAs interact directly with users, providing a conversational interface for accessing information, performing tasks, and facilitating communication. These digital entities understand speech, process requests, and provide responses or actions based on their programming and access to relevant systems. The benefits of VAs include improved patient care, enhanced efficiency, and better resource management.

VAs utilize advanced natural language processing to understand and respond to user queries conversationally, allowing for intuitive interactions. These assistants provide multi-platform accessibility, enabling users to access them through various devices such as smartphones, tablets, computers, and smart speakers. VA's personalization allows them customized responses and recommendations based on user profiles and previous patient interactions. They are built with robust integration capabilities to function effectively alongside electronic health record systems, scheduling systems, and other healthcare IT infrastructure. Many VAs also employ machine learning algorithms, enabling them to improve their performance continuously based on user interactions.

VAs, using natural language processing, empower patients and healthcare professionals by making it easier to obtain information or perform tasks without navigating complex interfaces. The ability to process and generate human-like speech enables these assistants to engage in more natural, context-aware conversations, improving the quality of automated interactions. This user-friendly interface enhances VAs' acceptance by healthcare professionals and patients, making users more comfortable interacting with them and instilling a sense of control and confidence, making the healthcare experience more reassuring.

VAs integrate seamlessly with healthcare IT infrastructure, including electronic health records, laboratory information, and pharmacy management systems. Advanced VAs offer multi-modal interactions, combining voice, text, and visual inputs and outputs. This versatility makes them accessible to users with different preferences or abilities, providing richer, more comprehensive engagement.

Extensive knowledge bases that include medical information, clinical guidelines, drug databases, and institutional policies inform and guide VAs. Accessing and synthesizing large amounts of medical knowledge enables these assistants to provide up-to-date, evidence-based information to clinicians and patients, supporting better decision-making and patient education.

VAs automate routine tasks such as scheduling appointments, sending reminders, filling out forms, and updating records. This automation saves time and allows clinicians to better interact with patients and focus on their clinical needs, thereby improving patient-clinician interaction and reducing their administrative burden.

Patient Care Skills

In 1986, Lawrence Rabiner published *A Tutorial on Hidden Markov Models and Selected Applications in Speech Recognition,* a landmark paper that revolutionized speech recognition technology. Rabiner's work provided a comprehensive mathematical framework for using Hidden Markov Models to analyze and interpret speech patterns. This approach became the foundation for many advancements in speech recognition, enabling systems to handle variability in pronunciation, accents, and noise. The principles he outlined remain integral to the voice recognition technology powering modern VAs, setting the stage for today's AI-driven interactions between humans and machines.

Patient-facing VAs facilitate a wide range of services to enhance patient care. These VAs handle appointment scheduling and reminders, ensuring patients do not miss important medical visits and arrive prepared with pre-visit information. They assist with medication management, supporting patients with dosage information, reminders, and potential side effect warnings. VAs educate patients by providing tailored descriptions and explanations of medical terms and procedures customized for each patient, making patients better informed and more engaged.

These assistants help track symptoms and vital signs for patients with chronic conditions, providing personalized management plans and lifestyle modification suggestions. They also support telemedicine initiatives by facilitating video consultations and assisting with post-consultation tasks such as medication refills or follow-up appointments. VAs augment mental health professionals by offering cognitive behavioral therapy exercises and mindfulness techniques while monitoring whether a patient requires intervention by a human mental health professional.

Clinician-facing VAs enhance efficiency and decision-making. They offer clinical decision support, providing quick access to relevant medical information, guidelines, and potential treatment options. They assist with clinical documentation, helping clinicians efficiently input and retrieve patient information. VAs contribute to workflow optimization and task management, allowing healthcare professionals to prioritize their work and manage their time more effectively. Medical researchers leverage VAs to perform more comprehensive literature searches and summarize findings.

Administrative VAs support business operations by automating various activities. These include:

Streamlines Claim Processing: Reduces errors and accelerates reimbursement cycles.

Inventory Management: Ensures that medical supplies and equipment are adequately stocked and efficiently utilized.

Staff Scheduling and Resource Allocation: Optimizes workforce and equipment utilization.

Regulatory Compliance: Monitor changes in regulations and reimbursement rules.

As healthcare organizations implement VAs to enhance efficiency and patient care, questions inevitably arise about the impact of this automation on the healthcare workforce. Understanding the relationship between digital and human workers becomes crucial for successfully utilizing these technologies.

Sidebar: Will Digital Workers Replace Human Workers?

Digital workers, including VAs, are replacing human workers, and this trend is rapidly accelerating. Like the introduction of other disruptive technologies, such as electric motors, word-processing software, and robotics, new jobs are being created.

Digital workers are already automating repetitive or routine tasks, such as data entry or assembly line work. However, specific tasks still require human creativity, problem-solving, and emotional intelligence, which digital workers cannot currently replicate. Jobs that involve management, interpersonal communication, and creative problem-solving are unlikely to be fully automated.

Even as digital workers become more prevalent, human oversight is crucial. Human workers must design, program, and monitor these digital systems, ensuring they function correctly and make ethical decisions. This human oversight is not just a necessity but a testament to the value and integral role of human workers in the era of digital transformation as we further digitize work.

While digital workers may replace some human jobs, individuals must continue developing their skills and stay current with new technologies. New skills will ensure they can meet the demands of the new jobs AI creates.

Implementation and Management of VAs

In 1991, the National Library of Medicine launched the *Unified Medical Language System* (UMLS), a ground-breaking initiative that created the first comprehensive thesaurus and ontology of biomedical terms. The UMLS unified various medical vocabularies, providing a standardized framework for representing and organizing complex healthcare terminology. This standardization became a cornerstone for accurate communication and interoperability across diverse healthcare systems. For virtual assistants (VAs) and healthcare AI, the UMLS plays a vital role in understanding, processing, and contextualizing medical conversations. Bridging linguistic gaps enhances AI-driven tools' ability to support clinicians and patients with precise information exchange.

Healthcare demands that VAs maintain high levels of accuracy and reliability in their responses and actions. Delivering trusted responses requires regular updates to the VA's knowledge base to ensure that the information they provide is current and evidence-based. Thorough testing protocols should be in place to validate the accuracy of VA responses across a wide range of scenarios.

The successful implementation of VAs depends heavily on user acceptance. Patients and healthcare professionals should be educated on VA capabilities and limitations to foster trust and encourage adoption. Organizations must provide comprehensive training programs to help users effectively interact with and leverage these tools. This education includes hands-on training sessions, user guides, and ongoing support to address questions or concerns. It is important to emphasize that VAs augment human capabilities rather than replace healthcare professionals and directly address concerns about job displacement or depersonalization of care.

Future VAs will incorporate more advanced emotional intelligence capabilities to understand better and respond to users' emotional states. This enhancement will benefit mental health counseling, enabling VAs to provide more empathetic and personalized support.

Integrating VAs with augmented reality (AR) technologies can guide healthcare professionals through complex procedures, offering real-time visual assistance. These advanced assistants also provide interactive 3D visualizations to help patients better understand their conditions and treatment options.

VAs adapt to diverse linguistic and cultural contexts, reflecting the needs of diverse populations. Future iterations will offer seamless multilingual support and culturally sensitive interactions, improving acceptance and accessibility across various patient populations.

The evolution of VAs mirrors broader advances in AI, particularly in systems capable of complex reasoning and decision-making. In my next *Bedside Consult*, I consider the future value of these technologies. The development of OpenAI's Q^* algorithm raises intriguing questions about the capacity of AI systems to engage in sophisticated medical reasoning and thought experiments—capabilities that could fundamentally transform how we approach clinical decision-making and medical research.

Bedside Consult: Understanding OpenAI's Q*— Are Computers Capable of Thought Experiments?

The development of OpenAI's Q* algorithm, described in Shelly Palmer's (2023) blog post *Understanding OpenAI's Rumored Humanity-Ending Algorithm*, presents a groundbreaking advancement in AI. While still in the realm of speculation, this development has significant implications for the future of clinical medicine and clinical research, particularly in precision and personalized medical care.

Q*, a combination of Q-learning and the Maryland Refutation Proof Procedure system, represents a major step toward *artificial general intelligence*. It employs Q-learning, a subset of reinforcement learning, enabling AI to make decisions autonomously. Unlike current reinforcement learning, which requires human feedback, Q-learning operates without human intervention.

This mirrors the human learning process, where trial and error play a crucial role. This advanced form of AI can understand, learn, and apply intelligence across various tasks akin to human capabilities. This capability means an AI system that can autonomously learn and adapt to complex medical environments in healthcare. AI systems could independently develop strategies for diagnosing diseases or recommending treatments, learning from vast datasets— and conducting thought experiments—without direct human intervention.

Accelerated Trial and Error

The autonomous decision-making ability of Q* could revolutionize diagnostics and treatment planning. AI systems could analyze patient data, consider a range of possible diagnoses, and suggest the most effective treatments based on learning from its simulations. This knowledge would improve the accuracy of diagnoses and tailor treatments to individual patient needs, a cornerstone of personalized medicine. Q* driven algorithms can create predictive disease progression and treatment outcomes models. These models are particularly beneficial in chronic diseases, where understanding the disease trajectory is crucial for effective management.

The trial-and-error aspect of Q-learning offers many additional clinical research paths. AI systems can simulate numerous scenarios or treatment outcomes, learning from each iteration. This approach accelerates drug discovery, optimizes treatment protocols, and predicts patient responses to various treatments, leading to more personalized care.

Advancing Discovery and Innovation

AI's ability to learn from trial and error without human input will accelerate clinical research. AI could autonomously design and simulate clinical trials, analyze results, and learn from each iteration, identifying the most promising treatments or understanding complex disease mechanisms more rapidly.

The advent of Q* aligns perfectly with the goals of personalized and precision medicine—to provide the right treatment to the right patient at the right time. By integrating and analyzing diverse data types, including genomic, environmental, and lifestyle factors, Q* can identify the most effective treatments for individual patients, enhancing the quality of care. This capability improves patient outcomes and reduces the trial-and-error approach often seen in current medical practices.

Ethical Considerations

While the anticipated benefits of Q* in healthcare are immense, it is crucial to approach its integration cautiously. Data privacy, ethical use of AI, and the possibility of AI misalignment with human values must be addressed. Ensuring that moral principles and regulations guide the use of such advanced AI systems in healthcare is paramount.

The speculated capabilities of OpenAI's Q* algorithm hold immense potential for transforming clinical medicine and research. By enhancing diagnostic accuracy, personalizing treatment plans, and revolutionizing drug discovery and clinical trials, Q* could significantly improve patient outcomes and the efficiency of healthcare delivery. However, as we navigate this exciting yet uncharted territory, balancing optimism with a healthy dose of caution is essential to ensure that the benefits of such technology are realized responsibly and ethically.

The journey of healthcare VAs—from basic voice recognition systems to sophisticated AI-powered clinical supports—represents a remarkable fusion of technological innovation and patient care. As these systems evolve, incorporating advances in emotional intelligence, AR, and complex reasoning capabilities will further transform healthcare delivery. However, the success of this transformation depends not just on technological sophistication but on our ability to integrate these tools thoughtfully into clinical practice, maintaining the essential human elements of patient care while leveraging technology to enhance efficiency and quality of care.

Virtual assistants are powerful enablers of a more accessible, efficient, and personalized healthcare system. Their ability to bridge gaps in care delivery, support clinical decision-making, and reduce administrative burden positions them as crucial tools in addressing healthcare's most pressing challenges. The continued evolution of these systems, guided by careful attention to ethics, privacy, and the preservation of human relationships, promises to enhance further their role in improving health outcomes.

PART II

Creating Tomorrow's Healthcare: AI Strategies

In Part I, we explored the fundamental concepts of healthcare artificial intelligence (AI), examining how these technologies reshape clinical practice through multimodal applications, predictive analytics, and augmented human expertise. As we move into Part II, I guide you through the strategic approaches critical for healthcare organizations to successfully implement and maintain AI systems while ensuring the delivery of quality care.

During my career, I witnessed firsthand how technology can dramatically transform research, improve quality and safety, drive economic efficiency, create new professional opportunities, and disrupt healthcare economics. However, I also saw how inadequate planning and implementation undermines even the most promising technology initiatives. The chapters ahead address these crucial aspects of healthcare AI deployment that often determine the difference between success and failure.

We begin by examining AI's revolutionary impact on healthcare research. From accelerating clinical trials and drug discovery to enhancing medical education and modernizing risk adjustment models, AI is fundamentally changing how we develop, validate, and apply medical knowledge. The introduction of systems like *Alpha-Fold* demonstrates AI's potential to unlock new understanding of biology, while AI-powered clinical trial matching and synthetic data generation are making research more efficient and cost-effective.

Quality and safety remain paramount in healthcare, and AI offers unprecedented opportunities to enhance both. I share insights into how organizations can leverage AI systems to improve patient safety, reduce medical errors, and ensure consistent, high-quality care delivery. Drawing from Donabedian's enduring structure, process, and outcomes model, we explore how AI can systematically strengthen our ability to monitor and enhance healthcare quality while maintaining essential human oversight.

The economic implications of healthcare AI cannot be overlooked. We examine how AI transforms clinical documentation, revenue cycle management, and operational efficiency. From reducing administrative burden through AI-enhanced electronic health record systems to optimizing resource utilization and improving revenue capture, understanding these economic factors is crucial for healthcare leaders to make strategic decisions about AI adoption.

The transformation of healthcare roles through AI represents both challenge and opportunity. We explore how AI creates new positions while reshaping traditional clinical and administrative functions. Just as the Industrial Revolution transformed manufacturing and word processing revolutionized office work, AI catalyzes the evolution of healthcare careers. Success requires healthcare organizations to balance technological advancement with human expertise, ensuring AI augments rather than replaces humans in patient care.

Finally, we examine the critical challenges of protecting patient privacy and ensuring cybersecurity in the age of AI. Recent high-profile incidents have shown that these considerations are more important than ever. I guide you through the essential strategies for protecting patient data while leveraging AI's capabilities, drawing on lessons learned from recent security breaches and emerging best practices in healthcare data protection.

Throughout Part II, I focus on practical, actionable insights that healthcare leaders can apply in their organizations. The challenges and opportunities we explore are not theoretical—they represent the current reality healthcare organizations must navigate as they implement AI technologies. I aim to provide you with the knowledge and frameworks needed to make informed decisions about AI implementation while avoiding common pitfalls and ensuring these powerful technologies serve their ultimate purpose: improving patient care.

As we delve into these advanced topics, remember that successful AI implementation requires a holistic approach that considers the technology and its impact on people, processes, and organizational culture. The chapters ahead will help you develop this comprehensive perspective, building on the foundational knowledge established in Part 1 to create a complete understanding of what it takes to succeed with AI in healthcare.

Join me as we explore these crucial aspects of healthcare AI and learn how to navigate the challenges and opportunities that lie ahead in this rapidly evolving field. Artificial intelligence is shaping the future of healthcare, and your understanding of these technologies is crucial in leading this transformation.

CHAPTER 8

AI in Healthcare Research

In 1747, aboard the HMS *Salisbury*, Scottish physician James Lind conducted what is widely regarded as the first controlled clinical trial in medical history. At the time, scurvy was a devastating illness among sailors, often leading to death during long voyages. Lind, determined to find a cure, selected 12 sailors suffering from scurvy and divided them into pairs. Each group received a different treatment, including cider, vinegar, seawater, and citrus fruits. Lind discovered that those given oranges and lemons recovered quickly, identifying a link between scurvy and dietary deficiencies, particularly a lack of vitamin C. This methodical approach to testing treatments established the foundation for evidence-based medicine, revolutionizing medical research. Lind's work demonstrated the importance of systematic experimentation, controlled variables, and reproducible results—principles that continue to shape clinical trials and medical advancements to this day.

Clinical trials are essential for advancing medical knowledge and developing new therapies. However, traditional clinical trial processes need help with participant recruitment, data management, and operational efficiency. Artificial intelligence (AI) offers numerous opportunities to transform clinical trials and accelerate the development of life-saving treatments.

AI-generated hypotheses guide the design and analysis of clinical trials. By identifying patient subgroups or treatment effect modifiers, AI can inform the selection of trial participants, the stratification of randomization, and the pre-specification of subgroup analyses. This focused selection leads to more targeted and efficient clinical trials, increasing the likelihood of detecting treatment benefits and adverse side effects.

AI streamlines participant recruitment by analyzing large datasets, such as electronic health records (EHRs) and patient registries, to identify eligible participants based on specific inclusion and exclusion criteria. Natural language processing (NLP) automates the extraction of relevant information from unstructured data sources, reducing the need for manual review and improving the speed and accuracy of adjudication. Pharmaceutical companies use this output from NLP and AI to match patients to their clinical trials based on eligibility criteria, reducing recruitment timelines and increasing patient enrollment rates.

Machine learning (ML) algorithms can generate computable phenotypes—digital representations of patient characteristics—which further help match trial participants with suitable clinical trials.

Improving data quality and completeness is essential for accurate and reliable results in clinical trials. AI helps automate data validation and error detection. ML algorithms identify inconsistencies, missing values, and outliers in clinical trial data, enabling researchers to address data quality issues proactively. By improving data quality and completeness, AI enhances the reliability of research findings and ensures that clinical trials are based on solid evidence.

AI can create synthetic data—new data generated based on learned patterns—which will revolutionize clinical trial operations. Synthetic data are computer-generated patient profiles that mimic real-world patient characteristics. Combining trial participant data with synthetic data expands the available research database, reducing the need for large and expensive control groups, making clinical trials more efficient. Additionally, AI can assist protocol optimization by simulating different trial designs and predicting their outcomes, helping researchers identify the most promising designs and minimizing the risk of failure.

Using AI in clinical trials raises important regulatory and ethical considerations. Regulatory agencies, such as the U.S. Food and Drug Administration, continually update guidance documents to ensure AI's safe and responsible deployment in clinical research. These guidelines address algorithm transparency, data privacy, and bias mitigation. Ethical considerations include ensuring that AI algorithms do not perpetuate or amplify health disparities. Deployed effectively, AI helps address potential disparities by ensuring that recruitment and analysis methods are inclusive and representative of diverse patient populations.

While AI's impact on clinical trials represents a significant advancement in healthcare research, equally revolutionary changes are occurring at the molecular level, where AI is transforming our understanding of the fundamental building blocks of life.

SideBar: Impact of AlphaFold and AlphaFold 3

AlphaFold, an AI system developed by Google DeepMind, revolutionized protein structure prediction. Proteins are the building blocks of life, and understanding their three-dimensional structures is crucial for advancing our knowledge of disease mechanisms, drug discovery, and biotechnology. AlphaFold uses deep learning algorithms to predict protein structures based on their amino acid sequences, achieving unprecedented accuracy in predicting the 3D shapes of proteins.

Building on the success of AlphaFold, *AlphaFold 3* expands upon its predecessor by predicting protein structures and modeling the interactions between proteins and small molecules. This latest iteration represents a significant step toward understanding the complex interplay between proteins and other molecules within biological systems. By accurately predicting how proteins interact with small molecules, AlphaFold 3 will revolutionize drug discovery processes, inspiring researchers with the promise of identifying and optimizing drug candidates more efficiently.

The impact of AlphaFold and AlphaFold 3 extends beyond their immediate applications in protein structure prediction and drug discovery. These AI systems demonstrate the power of AI in solving complex scientific problems and highlight the potential for AI to accelerate discovery and innovation across multiple domains in healthcare and life sciences.

Creative Ideation

In 1945, Vannevar Bush, an influential American engineer and science administrator, published a groundbreaking essay in *The Atlantic* titled "As We May Think." Written at the end of World War II, the essay called for redirecting scientific efforts toward advancing knowledge and improving human society. Central to Bush's vision was a revolutionary concept: the *Memex*, a desk-sized machine he imagined as a tool for augmenting human intellect. The Memex would allow users to store, retrieve, and cross-reference vast amounts of information, mimicking the associative processes of human memory. Bush envisioned it as an extension of the human mind, enabling users to link related ideas and generate new insights by organizing information into personalized *trails of thought*. Although the Memex was never built, it foreshadowed many modern innovations, including hypertext, personal computing, and the internet. Bush's prescient vision of human-machine collaboration for knowledge discovery finds its modern expression in artificial intelligence (AI) systems that analyze healthcare data, identify patterns, and generate novel hypotheses.

Like Bush's Memex, AI can empower healthcare professionals to ideate innovative approaches to patient care, operational efficiency, and medical research. For instance, by analyzing large and diverse datasets, AI algorithms identify patterns, relationships, and anomalies that may not be readily apparent to human observers. These insights inspire new research questions and hypotheses, guiding further investigation and discovery. In addition, AI helps discover new drug candidates by using deep learning algorithms to analyze millions of molecular structures and identify promising compounds for further investigation.

AI can generate hypotheses by detecting missingness and anomalies in clinical data. Missingness refers to the absence of essential data elements or variables in a dataset, which can be informative. For example, the consistent lack of data on social determinants of health in EHRs may indicate systemic biases or gaps in data collection practices. By identifying patterns of missingness, AI highlights areas where improvements in data quality and completeness are needed.

Anomalies refer to data points or patterns that deviate significantly from the norm. These anomalies may represent rare or previously unknown clinical phenotypes, adverse events, or treatment responses. By detecting anomalies in large datasets, AI can uncover new disease subtypes, drug side effects, or patient subpopulations that warrant further investigation.

AI-powered chatbots and virtual assistants serve as ideation partners for healthcare professionals, providing on-demand access to relevant information, suggesting alternative approaches to problem-solving, and facilitating brainstorming sessions.

As AI transforms how we conduct research and generate knowledge, it simultaneously revolutionizes how we share and teach that knowledge across healthcare.

Personalized Learning

In 1924, Sidney Pressey at Ohio State University pioneered the first automated teaching machine. This typewriter-like device could present questions, accept student responses, and provide immediate feedback through a mechanical scoring system. A century later, this early vision of personalized, machine-guided learning evolved into sophisticated AI-powered educational platforms that adapt content, assess performance, and simulate complex clinical scenarios. While Pressey's machine only tracked simple right-wrong answers, today's AI systems analyze nuanced learning patterns, provide detailed feedback, and create individualized learning pathways.

AI revolutionizes healthcare education by enabling personalized learning, adaptive assessment, and scalable knowledge dissemination. By leveraging ML algorithms and NLP, AI-powered educational platforms tailor content and instructional strategies to individual learners' needs, preferences, and performance, opening up exciting possibilities for the future of medical education.

Advances in healthcare education include AI-driven intelligent tutoring systems (ITS). These systems use AI algorithms to provide real-time feedback, guidance, and support to learners as they progress through educational content. ITS adapts to learners' knowledge levels, learning styles, and pace, ensuring each individual receives a customized learning experience.

AI can also create virtual patient simulations. These simulations use AI algorithms to generate realistic patient scenarios, allowing learners to practice clinical decision-making and problem-solving skills in a safe and controlled environment. They expose learners to a wide range of clinical cases, including rare or complex conditions, and provide immediate feedback on their performance. These simulations accelerate learning and ensure clinicians experience all the cases required to become competent in their field of study.

AI also facilitates the development of adaptive assessments that dynamically adjust question difficulty based on learners' responses. Adaptive assessments use ML algorithms to analyze learners' performance data to provide more accurate and efficient evaluations of knowledge and skills. Furthermore, AI-powered VAs provide on-demand access to medical knowledge and support for healthcare professionals and patients, enabling targeted learning.

Risk models are crucial in healthcare decision-making, resource allocation, and population health management. However, traditional risk models, such as the Centers for Medicare & Medicaid Services Hierarchical Condition Category model, often struggle to capture the full spectrum of variation in observed healthcare costs and outcomes. There is a growing need for the modernization of risk adjustment approaches to address the limitations of traditional risk models,

This modernization involves incorporating ML techniques, such as random forests, gradient boosting, and deep learning, to improve the accuracy and flexibility of risk prediction. ML algorithms can handle large and complex datasets, automatically detect patterns and interactions among variables, and model nonlinear relationships between risk factors and outcomes. By leveraging the power of ML, risk adjustment models better capture the heterogeneity of patient populations and provide more accurate predictions of healthcare costs and outcomes.

Modernizing risk adjustment models also involves incorporating social determinants of health (SDOH) data, such as income, education, and housing status. SDOH factors significantly impact healthcare outcomes and costs but are often not included in traditional risk models. By integrating SDOH data into risk adjustment approaches, healthcare organizations can better identify and address health disparities and allocate resources to populations with the greatest need.

Secondary Effects

While AI's primary applications in healthcare research focus on improving patient care, accelerating drug discovery, and enhancing medical education, it is essential to consider the secondary implications of AI use. These implications impact various stakeholders, from patients and healthcare providers to researchers and policymakers.

While healthcare AI can improve the efficiency and accuracy of medical decision-making, it may also alter patient-provider relationships. For example, using VAs for patient communication may reduce face-to-face time between patients and providers but help patients better understand their illness.

While AI can identify and address health inequities by analyzing large datasets and identifying underserved populations, it can also perpetuate or exacerbate existing biases if not carefully designed and implemented.

Ensuring the secure and ethical handling of patient data is critical for maintaining public trust and supporting the responsible use of AI.

Automating specific tasks improves healthcare efficiency but may also displace or alter the roles of specific healthcare professionals. Addressing these workforce implications and ensuring the appropriate training and use of AI in care delivery is crucial for realizing the full benefits of these technologies.

Interoperability, the ability of different systems and devices to exchange and interpret shared data, remains a crucial obstacle in developing robust AI tools and successfully integrating them into existing healthcare information technology. While the healthcare industry generates vast amounts of data from various sources, including EHR systems, medical imaging, wearable devices, and genomic databases, this data often exists in silos categorized by incompatible semantics, making it challenging to develop and deploy AI algorithms.

The successful implementation of AI in healthcare research depends on the effective collaboration between human expertise and AI. My next *Bedside Consult* explores this synergy, which demonstrates how technology and human knowledge can work together to advance patient care.

Bedside Consult: Collaborative Intelligence—How Human Expertise and AI Synergize in Healthcare

AI holds immense potential to revolutionize healthcare by improving patient outcomes, reducing costs, and optimizing clinical processes. However, realizing this promise requires a thoughtful approach to developing AI models, particularly regarding the quality and curation of training data. As healthcare executives navigate the rapidly evolving landscape of AI, understanding the crucial role of human expertise in this process is essential to evaluating and choosing which AI applications are appropriate for their organization.

The training data is at the heart of any successful AI implementation. These datasets, often comprising patient records, clinical notes, and medical images, form the foundation upon which AI models learn to make predictions and recommendations. However, raw healthcare data is often complex, heterogeneous, and biased. With proper curation and annotation by subject matter experts, AI models can avoid perpetuating inaccuracies and biases that could negatively impact patient care.

Clinicians, researchers, and other domain experts possess the knowledge and experience to evaluate training data's relevance, quality, and representativeness. By carefully selecting, cleaning, and annotating datasets, these experts ensure that AI models learn from accurate, unbiased, and clinically meaningful information.

Leverage Human Expertise to Enhance AI Systems

Organizations can leverage human expertise to curate data for AI training in various ways. One approach is establishing multidisciplinary guideline development groups with representatives from diverse clinical specialties, geographic regions, and patient populations. These groups can collaborate to define the scope and purpose of the AI model, identify relevant data sources, and establish criteria for data inclusion and exclusion.

The process of annotation, which involves labeling and categorizing data to provide context and meaning for AI models, remains a critical aspect of data creation. Human annotators, often subject matter experts, employ techniques such as named entity recognition to identify key clinical concepts, sentiment analysis to capture the emotional tone of the text, and dependency parsing to understand the relationships between words. These tasks require an expert understanding of medical terms, clinical workflows, administrative workflows, and the nuances of patient care—knowledge that only experienced healthcare professionals can provide.

Organizations can recruit content experts through various channels, including professional networks and partnerships with academic institutions, or outsource the work to existing clinical content development organizations. It is essential to ensure that annotators have the necessary domain expertise and are trained in the organization's specific annotation guidelines and quality control processes.

Ongoing Feedback

Human experts' involvement extends beyond the initial data preparation phase. As AI models are developed and refined, ongoing feedback from clinicians and other stakeholders is essential to validate the model's outputs and ensure their alignment with clinical best practices. This iterative process of evaluation and refinement, guided by human expertise, is crucial to building safe, effective, and trustworthy AI systems.

Reinforcement learning from human feedback (RLHF) represents a promising approach to incorporating human expertise in AI development. RLHF is an innovative technique that involves training AI models through interactions with human evaluators who provide feedback on the model's outputs. This approach allows the model to learn from the knowledge and judgment of domain experts, ensuring that the AI system aligns with clinical best practices, patient safety, and ethical considerations.

Applying RLHF

RLHF is applied in several ways to enhance the quality and relevance of healthcare AI models. For example, clinicians provide feedback on the model's diagnostic or treatment recommendations, helping the AI system learn to make more accurate and con-text-appropriate decisions for clinician users. Similarly, patient representatives offer insights into the usability and acceptability of patient-centric AI-powered tools, ensuring that they meet the needs and preferences of the patient end-users.

Reward modeling offers a specific technique that is valuable within RLHF. Human evaluators rank or rate the model's outputs based on their quality or appropriateness. The model then learns to predict these rewards and adjusts its behavior to maximize the predicted rewards. This approach enables the AI system to learn complex tasks, such as providing empathetic patient communication or adapting to individual patient needs, which are difficult to define with simple objective functions.

Comparative ranking is another RLHF technique in which human evaluators rank multiple AI-generated outputs based on their relative quality or suitability. The model then learns to produce outputs consistently ranked higher by the evaluators. This method helps the AI system understand the nuances and contextual factors influencing clinical decision-making, leading to more refined and appropriate recommendations.

Build Multidisciplinary Teams for AI Projects

Healthcare executives must also consider the importance of diversity and inclusivity when assembling teams to work on AI projects. Guideline development groups, for example, should be multidisciplinary and include representatives from various clini-cal specialties, geographic regions, and patient populations. This diversity of perspectives helps developers train AI models on data that reflects the broad spectrum of patient needs, experiences, and cultural differences.

Transparency and collaboration are equally critical in the development of healthcare AI. Organizations must establish clear processes for documenting data sources, annotation techniques, and model performance metrics. Sharing this information with regulatory bodies, healthcare providers, and patients helps build trust in AI systems and facilitates safe and effective deployment in clinical settings.

Learning From CPG Processes

Furthermore, healthcare organizations can draw valuable lessons from the established processes to develop clinical practice guidelines (CPGs). CPGs are researched statements developed by subject matter expert teams that provide recommendations for clinical care based on the best available evidence. The development of CPGs involves rigorous evidence synthesis, multidisciplinary expert input, and stakeholder consultation. Applying similar principles to the development of AI models helps ensure that they are grounded in the best available evidence and aligned with clinical best practices.

As the healthcare industry continues to embrace AI, executives should prioritize the role of human expertise in every stage of the development process. By investing in multidisciplinary teams, fostering collaboration, and ensuring transparency, organizations can harness the power of AI to transform patient care while mitigating potential risks and biases. The path forward requires a thoughtful, human-centered approach that recognizes the indispensable value of clinical knowledge and experience in shaping the future of healthcare AI.

The development of AI for healthcare is not purely technical; it is deeply human. The expertise of clinicians, researchers, and other subject matter experts is essential to curating high-quality training data, guiding the development of AI models, and ensuring their safe and effective deployment in clinical settings. By prioritizing human expertise, collaboration, and innovative approaches like RLHF, healthcare organizations can unlock the transformative capacity of AI to improve patient outcomes, optimize clinical processes, and drive innovation in healthcare delivery. As healthcare executives navigate this exciting frontier, keeping human expertise at the center of AI development will be the key to success.

Integrating artificial intelligence into healthcare research marks a pivotal moment in medical history, comparable to the introduction of the microscope or the discovery of X-rays. As we continue to develop and refine these technologies, the partnership between human expertise and AI will remain central to advancing medical knowledge and improving patient care. The future of healthcare research lies not in choosing between human insight and AI but in leveraging their unique strengths to create more effective, efficient, and equitable healthcare systems.

CHAPTER 9

Enhancing Quality and Safety

In 1904, Dr. Ernest Amory Codman began work on the *End Result System*, the first systematic attempt to track patient outcomes and evaluate healthcare quality. Codman's revolutionary approach involved following each patient's case to identify successes and failures in treatment, establishing the foundation for modern healthcare quality measurement. More than a century later, artificial intelligence (AI) transformed Codman's vision, enabling healthcare organizations to analyze millions of patient outcomes in real time and proactively improve care quality.

To explore AI's potential to transform healthcare, we must ground our discussion in a comprehensive understanding of healthcare quality. Avedis Donabedian's *Donabedian Model* provides an excellent framework for this purpose. This model, a cornerstone in healthcare quality assessment for decades, offers valuable insights into how we can integrate AI into healthcare to enhance care quality and patient safety.

Donabedian's model consists of three interconnected components: *structure*, *process*, and *outcomes*. Each plays a vital role in shaping healthcare quality and offers unique opportunities for AI integration.

Structure: The Foundation of AI-Enabled Healthcare

Structure encompasses the organizational and environmental factors that influence healthcare delivery. It includes the foundational elements necessary to implement and utilize AI technologies effectively. A robust structural framework begins with comprehensive data management systems and interoperable electronic health record (EHR) systems. These systems are the backbone for AI applications, providing the necessary data for training models and generating insights.

Advanced analytics platforms and computing infrastructure form another crucial aspect of the structural component. These technologies enable healthcare organizations to process data efficiently and derive meaningful insights. Recent advancements in cloud and edge computing enhanced these capabilities, allowing for more efficient processing of large datasets and real-time analytics.

Equally important is the human element of the structural component. Healthcare organizations must employ skilled personnel to develop, implement, and manage AI systems. These qualified personnel include data scientists who design and train AI models, IT professionals who integrate these systems into existing infrastructure, and clinicians trained in AI who can aid development and effectively use these tools in patient care.

Process: AI-Enhanced Care Delivery

Process focuses on delivering healthcare services, including interactions between providers and patients and the procedures and protocols followed in care delivery. AI integration requires incorporating AI tools and insights into decision-making processes and clinical workflows.

To optimize AI's impact on care quality and safety, healthcare organizations must carefully design and implement AI-enabled processes that align with evidence-based guidelines, best practices, and effective clinical workflows. This involves establishing clear protocols for using AI in different care scenarios, including diagnostic support, treatment planning, and medication management. Organizations must train healthcare providers to effectively utilize AI insights and incorporate them into their clinical decision-making while maintaining human oversight.

Recent developments in process optimization include using AI-powered virtual assistants. These sophisticated tools guide healthcare providers through complex clinical pathways, ensuring adherence to best practices and reducing variability in care delivery. AI assistants help standardize care processes and improve quality by providing real-time, context-specific guidance.

Outcomes: Measuring AI's Impact

Outcomes assess the results and impact of healthcare services on patient health, quality of life, and overall well-being. This component evaluates the effectiveness of AI-enabled interventions in improving patient outcomes, reducing adverse events, and enhancing care quality and safety.

Organizations should establish clear metrics and performance indicators to assess AI's impact on healthcare outcomes. These include patient satisfaction, complications, readmission, and mortality rates. By continuously monitoring and analyzing these outcomes, healthcare organizations can identify areas where AI positively impacts care and areas that require further improvement or refinement of AI systems.

Recent advancements in AI enable more sophisticated outcome prediction models that can account for a broader range of factors, including social determinants of health and patient-reported outcomes. These models provide a more comprehensive view of the impact of AI interventions on patient health and well-being, allowing for more nuanced and personalized approaches to care.

While the Donabedian framework provides the structural foundation for understanding AI's role in healthcare quality, the practical application of AI in clinical settings demonstrates how these theoretical principles translate into tangible improvements in patient care. One of the most promising areas is clinical decision support, where AI directly enhances a healthcare provider's ability to deliver high-quality care.

Clinical Decision Support

In 1954, Paul Meehl published *Clinical Versus Statistical Prediction*, demonstrating how statistical methods could complement clinical judgment. This early work presaged AI-enabled clinical decision support. While Meehl is most known for arguing that statistical prediction methods generally outperform clinical judgment, his work did not suggest that statistical methods could not support clinical judgment. In contrast, he advocated using statistical information to inform and enhance clinical decision-making, not replace it entirely.

AI can enhance clinical decision-making and improve patient safety. By analyzing vast amounts of patient data, AI algorithms identify patterns and provide valuable insights to clinicians, empowering them to make more informed decisions.

AI helps healthcare providers focus on what is most important in clinical care by filtering through vast amounts of data and highlighting key insights and actionable patient-specific information. AI relieves healthcare professionals from information overload and time pressure, allowing them to prioritize and streamline decision-making.

For example, large language models now provide real-time assistance to clinicians by summarizing patient histories, suggesting differential diagnoses, and recommending evidence-based treatment options. These AI-powered assistants help clinicians quickly access relevant information and make more informed decisions, especially in complex cases or rare conditions. This assistance leads to personalized treatment recommendations, fewer medical errors, better patient outcomes, and reduced medical costs.

Recent developments in AI introduced more advanced context-aware systems. These systems adapt their recommendations based on the specific clinical scenario, patient preferences, and available clinical resources. For instance, in a scenario where a patient has multiple chronic conditions and is taking several medications, the AI system might recommend a treatment plan that minimizes drug interactions. These systems provide more nuanced guidance, helping clinicians navigate complex decision-making processes to deliver personalized medicine.

In addition, AI helps clinicians triage patient cases based on severity and urgency. AI can focus healthcare providers on the most critical cases by analyzing patient data, predicting the likelihood of adverse events or clinical deterioration, and allocating resources accordingly. This targeted approach ensures that patients receive timely and appropriate care, improving outcomes and reducing the risk of complications.

Human Oversight

While AI offers significant benefits in healthcare decision-making, it is essential to emphasize the importance of human oversight. AI is solely a tool to support and augment human expertise rather than replace clinical judgment. Healthcare professionals must remain actively involved in the decision-making process, interpreting AI-generated insights and considering them in the context of individual patient needs and preferences. It is also important to acknowledge that AI has risks and limitations. These include biases in AI algorithms, data privacy concerns, and the need for continuous validation and updating of AI models. Understanding and addressing these challenges is crucial for AI's responsible and effective use in healthcare.

Establishing clear guidelines and protocols for using AI in clinical decision-making is also important. These guidelines include defining the roles and responsibilities of healthcare providers, ensuring transparency in AI algorithms, and establishing mechanisms for human oversight and intervention when necessary. By striking the right balance between AI-supported decision-making and human expertise, healthcare organizations can optimize the benefits of AI while maintaining the highest standards of patient care.

To be effective, healthcare professionals need to achieve *AI literacy* training. This training includes education in AI tools and understanding their limitations, biases, and the importance of critically evaluating AI-generated recommendations. Such education helps healthcare providers leverage AI effectively while maintaining clinical autonomy.

As AI continues to enhance clinical decision-making, its integration into patient monitoring systems represents another advancement in healthcare quality and safety. These monitoring applications demonstrate how AI augments human capabilities in real-time patient care settings.

Sidebar: Enabled Monitoring—From Vital Signs to Computer Vision

Integrating AI into patient monitoring led to the development of comprehensive systems that combine vital sign analysis, real-time alerts, and computer vision to provide a holistic approach to patient care. These systems address challenges traditional monitoring methods face, such as high rates of false alarms and missed early signs of clinical deterioration.

At the core of these AI-enabled systems is the continuous collection of monitoring data from medical device sensors. Advanced machine learning algorithms analyze this data in real time, establishing personalized baselines for each patient and detecting deviations from normal physiological parameters. This approach allows for the early identification of problems and alerts clinicians to intervene promptly to prevent adverse events.

These system capabilities extend beyond routine monitoring. In surgical care, AI-powered systems analyze data from additional sources, combining wound imaging with the details in the EHR. Computer vision and AI-assisted monitoring enhance patient safety using cameras and advanced image processing algorithms to monitor patient activity and behavior in clinical settings. For example, AI algorithms can analyze post-operative wound images using computer vision techniques to identify signs of inflammation, redness, or discharge. If concerning features are detected, the system alerts the surgical team and suggests treatment options, prompting timely intervention and preventing the progression of infection.

These systems can detect falls, monitor patient positioning, and identify changes in patient behavior that may indicate distress or deterioration. In intensive care units, AI-assisted monitoring systems use computer vision to monitor patient position, movement, and interaction with medical devices, such as ventilators or intravenous lines. These systems alert nurses to patient safety issues, enabling prompt intervention and preventing complications.

AI and computer vision advancements introduce sophisticated capabilities, including gait analysis for fall risk assessment and facial recognition for pain detection. When integrated into clinical workflows, these technologies improve the quality of care and enhance patient safety.

Integrating these monitoring approaches creates a more complete and nuanced understanding of patient health. These multimodal early warning systems allow for detecting subtle signs of deterioration that traditional monitoring methods miss.

Quality and Safety Surveillance

AI plays a pivotal role in revolutionizing healthcare quality and safety surveillance processes. Healthcare AI surveillance tools can continuously analyze system-wide care patterns using data from EHRs, claims databases, and administrative systems. By continuously analyzing vast amounts of aggregated patient data and care processes, AI-powered systems identify systemic areas for improvement, including workflow inefficiencies, variations in care quality, and safety risks across healthcare organizations.

For instance, an AI system might identify a pattern of increased complications associated with a particular surgical procedure across multiple facilities, prompting a review of protocols and exploring interventions to improve outcomes. This constant vigilance enables healthcare systems to maintain high standards of care and proactively address issues before they become widespread problems.

Furthermore, AI contributes to quality assurance by analyzing large datasets to identify the best practices and evidence-based guidelines. This analysis promotes standardization and consistency in healthcare delivery, ensuring patients receive optimal treatment regardless of facility or clinician. By highlighting variations in care and outcomes, AI-powered analytics guides targeted quality improvement initiatives and help healthcare organizations allocate resources more effectively.

While advances in AI-enabled monitoring and surveillance show great promise, healthcare can learn valuable lessons from other high-reliability industries that successfully implement systematic safety reporting. One industry offers a compelling model that has dramatically improved its safety record.

Lessons from Aviation

In 1960, commercial aviation experienced 67 accidents per million departures globally; by 2022, this rate had plummeted to approximately 1 accident per million departures. This dramatic improvement was not statistical. It represented thousands of lives saved.

In 1960, there were approximately 40 fatal accidents per year in commercial aviation; by 2022, despite a massive increase in air travel, fatal accidents had dropped to an average of 5 per year globally. This remarkable achievement stems mainly from the industry's long-standing commitment to error investigation, data analysis, and robust safety reporting, fostering a culture of continuous improvement and enhanced overall safety.

Healthcare providers can improve their ability to identify, analyze, and mitigate safety risks by adopting these principles, leveraging the power of AI, and addressing the challenges posed by the current malpractice legal environment.

Patient safety reporting systems are critical for identifying and addressing medical errors, near misses, and adverse events. These systems enable healthcare professionals to submit reports of incidents and concerns, allowing organizations to conduct root-cause analyses and implement systemic improvements to prevent future occurrences. However, traditional reporting systems often face challenges, including underreporting, lack of anonymity, and fear of retribution among staff members. The current legal environment for medical malpractice in the United States exacerbates this problem by fostering a culture of fear and defensiveness among healthcare providers.

To overcome these barriers, healthcare organizations can draw inspiration from the Aviation Safety Reporting System (ASRS), established in 1976 and managed by NASA. The ASRS allows aviation professionals, including pilots, flight attendants, and ground personnel, to submit confidential reports of safety incidents and concerns without fear of punishment or legal action. This system has been instrumental in identifying and addressing systemic safety issues in aviation, leading to significant improvements in safety practices and regulations.

Key features of the ASRS that healthcare organizations can adopt include:

- Confidentiality and anonymity
- Independent management
- A non-punitive approach
- Timely feedback and action

By ensuring that reports are de-identified and managed by an independent entity, healthcare professionals are more likely to report safety concerns openly and honestly. Emphasizing a non-punitive approach focused on learning and improvement rather than blame or punishment further encourages reporting and fosters a safety culture.

However, implementing such a system effectively in the United States requires addressing the monumental barrier posed by the current legal framework for medical malpractice. The fear of litigation and economic consequences creates a chilling effect on open reporting of errors and near-misses. To fully realize the benefits of a patient safety reporting system, advocating for and implementing legal reforms that support a culture of safety and learning is essential.

Critical areas for malpractice law reform to support effective patient safety reporting include:

Safe Harbor Provisions: These provisions implement legal protections for healthcare providers who report safety concerns in good faith, shielding them from using these reports in malpractice litigation.

Confidentiality Protections: Strengthening legal safeguards ensures that safety reports cannot be discovered or used as evidence in malpractice lawsuits, like protections afforded to aviation safety reports.

Apology Laws: Expand and strengthen laws that allow healthcare providers to express empathy and apologize to patients without these statements being used as admissions of liability in court.

Alternative Dispute Resolution: Encourage the use of mediation and other alternative dispute resolution mechanisms to address patient grievances without resorting to costly and adversarial litigation.

Caps on Non-economic Damages: Implement reasonable limits on non-economic damages in malpractice cases to reduce the fear of excessive financial penalties while ensuring fair patient compensation.

Administrative Compensation Systems: Explore using no-fault administrative compensation systems, such as workers' compensation programs, for specific medical injuries.

These reforms create an environment more conducive to open reporting and discussing safety issues. They allow healthcare organizations, supported by the federal and state governments, to implement effective patient safety reporting systems modeled after successful programs like the ASRS.

With a supportive legal framework, healthcare organizations can focus on implementing robust patient safety reporting systems. This implementation should include developing transparent reporting processes, ensuring confidentiality and anonymity, engaging independent management teams, fostering a non-punitive culture, providing timely feedback and action, and integrating with existing quality improvement processes.

AI can enhance the capabilities of these reporting systems. AI-powered analysis of safety reports offers several advantages:

Pattern Recognition: AI algorithms quickly sift through large volumes of reports to identify recurring themes or patterns that might indicate systemic issues.

Natural Language Processing (NLP): Advanced NLP techniques extract meaningful insights from unstructured text data, allowing for a more nuanced understanding of reported incidents and near-misses.

Predictive Analytics: By analyzing historical data and current trends, AI systems predict areas of increased risk, allowing for proactive measures.

Real-time Monitoring: AI-powered systems continuously monitor incoming reports, alerting relevant personnel to urgent safety concerns.

Automated Classification and Routing: AI helps categorize and route reports to appropriate departments or individuals for review and action.

Sentiment Analysis: AI analyzes the tone and sentiment of reports, potentially identifying areas of particular concern or frustration among staff or patients.

Cross-referencing With Other Data Sources: AI systems can integrate data from patient safety reports with other sources of information to provide a more comprehensive view of safety risks.

By implementing AI-enhanced patient safety reporting systems within a reformed legal framework, healthcare organizations create a more robust and responsive approach to identifying and mitigating safety risks. This technology-driven approach, combined with the lessons learned from the successful aviation reporting system and supported by a legal environment that encourages openness and learning, will greatly improve patient safety and the overall quality of care.

However, implementing AI in patient safety reporting systems should be done thoughtfully and ethically. Healthcare organizations must ensure that AI systems are transparent, explainable, and free from bias. They must also maintain human oversight to interpret AI-generated insights and make final decisions on safety interventions.

This comprehensive approach to patient safety, combining technological innovation with necessary legal and cultural changes, can transform healthcare delivery in the United States. It would improve outcomes, reduce medical errors and litigation costs, and increase trust between healthcare providers and their communities.

While AI technologies can help improve healthcare quality and safety, they also present new challenges in managing healthcare information. As our systems become more sophisticated in collecting and analyzing data, we must remain vigilant about the quality and accuracy of AI-generated information. The same tools that can enhance patient care can also, if misused, contribute to the spread of healthcare misinformation. My next *Bedside Consult* examines this critical challenge and provides practical guidance for healthcare professionals in protecting patients from AI-driven healthcare misinformation.

Bedside Consult: Protect Patients from AI-Driven Healthcare Misinformation

The proliferation of health misinformation, a complex and formidable issue, was underscored by a 2024 Supreme Court case involving the Biden administration's battle against false COVID-19 vaccine claims on social media. As a healthcare information technology and public health expert, I am deeply alarmed by the dangers of medical misinformation, mainly as AI becomes increasingly integrated into patient care, exacerbating the problem.

The New York Times's "Health Misinformation is Evolving. Here's How to Spot It" (Blum, 2024) offers valuable insights into the evolving nature of health misinformation. Blum points out that unsubstantiated health hacks, cures, and quick fixes have spread widely on social media, while conspiracy theories that fueled vaccine hesitancy during the COVID-19 pandemic are now undermining trust in vaccines against other diseases. Recent outbreaks of measles, previously deemed eradicated in the United States, are evidence of the impact of a reduction in childhood vaccinations fostered by misinformation. Rapid developments in AI make it even harder for people to distinguish between true and false information online.

Test AI-Generated Content

As AI integrates into patient care, it is imperative that organizations rigorously test the AI output for accuracy and regularly monitor it to prevent the dissemination of harmful misinformation. Equally crucial is educating doctors, nurses, other clinicians, and patients about the risks of healthcare AI misinformation and how to identify it. The primary threat to patient exposure to misinformation is the abundance of unverified and untrusted healthcare websites that mimic reputable institutions but can quickly disseminate AI-generated misinformation.

Identify Misinformation

Blum's article provides valuable tips for recognizing misinformation, such as looking out for unsubstantiated claims, emotional appeals, and *fake experts* who lack relevant medical credentials or expertise. It also recommends validating claims with multiple trusted sources, such as health agency websites, and tracking down the original source of information to check for omitted or altered details.

I fear that AI-generated misinformation will continue to be used to support political agendas, such as those proposed by anti-vaccination supporters who reject the proven science of the value of vaccinations. Additionally, unscrupulous drug or supplement manufacturers may offer unsubstantiated information about their products, prioritizing profit over patient health and safety.

As Blum's article rightly points out, addressing misinformation within personal circles necessitates empathy and patience. Using phrases like—*I understand*, and *it's challenging to discern who to trust*—can help maintain relationships while guiding individuals toward reliable resources. Local public health sites and university websites may be more effective for those distrusting national agencies.

Duty to Call-out Misinformation

As healthcare professionals and informed citizens, we must remain vigilant in identifying and addressing health misinformation, particularly as AI advances and complicates the information landscape. By educating ourselves and others about the risks of misinformation, validating claims with trusted sources, and engaging in empathetic dialogue, we can work together to protect patient health and safety in the face of this growing threat.

Using artificial intelligence in healthcare quality and safety systems represents more than technological advancement—it embodies the next evolution of Donabedian's enduring three-pillar model of structure, process, and outcomes. From AI-enhanced clinical decision support to sophisticated safety surveillance systems, we are witnessing the transformation of healthcare delivery. Yet, as our exploration of this transformation reveals, the most effective approach combines AI's power with human wisdom and oversight. Success requires thoughtful use of technology within existing quality outlines, robust safety reporting systems protected by appropriate legal reforms, and vigilant protection against misinformation. As we move forward, maintaining this balance between technological innovation and human judgment is critical in realizing the power of artificial intelligence to enhance healthcare quality and safety while preserving the essential human elements of care delivery.

CHAPTER 10

The Economics of Healthcare AI

In 1913, Henry Ford revolutionized manufacturing by introducing the *moving assembly line* at the Ford Motor Company. By breaking down automobile production into a series of standardized, repeatable tasks performed on a conveyor belt system, Ford reduced the production time of a Model T from 12 hours to an astonishing 93 minutes. This innovation made cars more affordable for the average consumer and transformed industrial practices worldwide, becoming a cornerstone of modern mass production. Just as Ford's assembly line enabled a new level of productivity and accessibility in the automotive industry, artificial intelligence (AI) driven innovations are enhancing efficiency, reducing costs, and improving patient outcomes in healthcare.

By assisting clinicians in image analysis, diagnosis, and treatment planning tasks, healthcare AI enables clinicians to see more patients while providing higher-quality care. Increasing clinician productivity translates into significant cost savings for healthcare organizations, payers, and patients.

In addition, AI helps optimize resource utilization and reduce waste by analyzing large datasets and identifying patterns. It assists healthcare organizations in making more informed decisions about resource allocation, supply chain management, and capacity planning, leading to more efficient resource use, reduced costs, and improved financial performance.

The economic impact of AI on healthcare is not limited to cost savings and market growth. AI can also disrupt traditional business models and reshape the competitive landscape for provider and payer organizations. For example, the increasing use of AI in telemedicine and remote monitoring enables new entrants to compete with established healthcare providers, leading to increased competition and lower prices.

AI is also driving innovation and growth in the healthcare technology sector. The increasing demand for AI-powered solutions creates new opportunities for startups, established technology companies, and healthcare organizations to develop and commercialize innovative products and services. Venture capital firms' recent interest in AI companies is leading to record funding levels for these companies.

While AI's economic potential spans many areas, none is more immediately impactful than its ability to address one of healthcare's most persistent challenges: the documentation burden placed on clinicians.

The Documentation Dilemma

Healthcare professionals spend a disproportionate amount of their workday on documentation tasks. This effort includes recording patient encounters, updating medical histories, and detailing treatment plans in electronic health records (EHRs). The time devoted to these administrative duties detracts from direct patient care, leading to decreased productivity and, more alarmingly, clinician burnout.

The current state of EHR systems exacerbates this issue. Most systems were designed to optimize documentation for billing purposes rather than enhance patient care. This misalignment adds an extra layer of complexity to the documentation process, further increasing documentation time and cognitive load placed on clinicians. While necessary for financial operations, the result is a system that often hinders rather than supports patient care.

AI-enhanced EHR systems can process and interpret clinical notes and other free-text data. Using natural language processing (NLP), these systems automatically identify essential information, such as patient symptoms, diagnoses, and treatment plans, and populate the relevant fields in the EHR.

Virtual scribes utilize NLP and real-time speech analysis to listen to patient-clinician conversations and generate accurate, comprehensive summaries of the encounter. By capturing essential details such as medical history, current symptoms, and prescribed medications, virtual scribes produce draft documentation that clinicians quickly review and modify before integrating into the patient's EHR.

By automating routine tasks and providing intelligent decision support, these systems improve patient care quality by minimizing errors associated with manual data entry and reducing the likelihood of missing or misinterpreted information. This improvement in data accuracy has far-reaching economic implications, from reducing costly medical errors to enhancing the efficiency of billing processes.

By automating routine tasks and providing intelligent decision support, AI can reduce clinician burnout, allowing clinicians to focus more on direct patient care. Burnout's economic impact results in reduced quality of care, increased medical errors, and a shortage of clinicians as professionals leave direct patient care roles.

Some provider organizations use AI-powered chatbots to interact with patients, gathering information about symptoms, medical history, and treatment adherence before the clinical encounter. These virtual assistants provide personalized health information, answer common questions, and triage patients based on the severity of their symptoms. By automating these tasks, chatbots reduce clinicians' workload, improve patient engagement, and reduce unnecessary clinic visits.

AI-enhanced EHR systems optimize the prescription process by automatically checking for compliance with a patient's health plan's formulary. The systems verify coverage, suggest alternative medications, and facilitate prior authorization.

AI also improves medication reconciliation. When hospitals discharge or transition patients between care settings, AI automatically compares the patient's current medication list with those prescribed during the recent encounter. The system identifies discrepancies, potential interactions, and duplicate therapies, providing the physician with a reconciled medication list for review and approval.

Need for Overhaul and Innovation in EHR Systems

The current generation of EHR systems needs to improve usability, flexibility, and adaptability to integrate emerging AI technologies. Many systems are built on inflexible legacy architectures that are difficult to navigate and ill-suited for integrating advanced technologies.

EHR systems must evolve to easily integrate new technologies without requiring major system overhauls or disruptions to patient care. Easy integration requires the development of plug-and-play architectures, microservices, and other modular approaches.

Achieving this level of EHR system innovation also requires changes in healthcare delivery's regulatory environment and vendor economic incentives. Current certification requirements for EHR systems act as barriers to innovation by focusing on compliance with narrow functional criteria rather than promoting flexibility and adaptability. Efforts to foster EHR system interoperability need to catch up with rapid technological changes, and entrenched EHR system vendors need to remove barriers to entry for innovative startup companies that threaten their monopoly power. Regulatory frameworks need to shift towards more outcome-based approaches that encourage innovation and the development of EHR systems that are user-friendly, interoperable, and capable of supporting advanced technologies.

The evolution of healthcare data systems, from paper records to AI-enhanced EHR systems, highlights the critical need for seamless data exchange and integration. As we examine the steps to achieve true interoperability, we must consider the technical and organizational challenges that healthcare organizations and system vendors face in achieving this goal.

Side Bar: Full Interoperability

The next generation of EHR systems requires a design that supports interoperability and full data exchange. Despite efforts to promote data exchange through initiatives like Health Information Exchanges (HIEs) and Fast Healthcare Interoperability Resources (FHIR) standards, many EHR systems remain siloed and fail to share data with other systems seamlessly. This data fragmentation hinders healthcare AI's ability to fully support patient care and learn from diverse patient populations to generate insights that improve outcomes.

Recent advances in cloud and edge computing technologies offer promising solutions for enhancing the flexibility and scalability of EHR systems. Recent developments, such as federated learning and differential privacy techniques, provide promising solutions to address data privacy concerns while still enabling the training of robust AI models.

Economic incentives for adopting and using the EHR systems need realignment to promote innovation and improved outcomes. Current reimbursement models prioritize volume over quality, discouraging the adoption of technologies that enhance patient care without increasing revenue. To overcome this challenge, policymakers and payers should develop new payment models that reward innovative technologies and prioritize patient outcomes over service volume.

AI-enhanced EHR systems are well-suited to support value-based care models, which tie reimbursement to quality of care rather than volume of services. By providing comprehensive patient data analysis and predictive modeling capabilities, these systems help healthcare organizations identify high-risk patients, implement targeted interventions, and track outcomes more effectively. Alignment with value-based care models leads to improved financial performance for healthcare providers and payers. It ensures that resources are directed towards improving patient outcomes while enhancing the overall efficiency of care delivery.

Clinical and Business Operations

In 1980, New Jersey pioneered the Diagnosis-Related Groups (DRGs) system, introducing the first prospective payment system in American healthcare. Starting with a small group of hospitals categorized by their budget positions, this three-year experiment eventually encompassed all New Jersey hospitals before becoming a national model. DRGs created standardized units of hospital activity with fixed pricing—a revolutionary concept that transformed healthcare economics and laid the groundwork for modern AI-driven revenue cycle management (RCM) systems.

Integrating AI into clinical operations offers substantial economic benefits alongside improvements in patient care. By leveraging vast amounts of data generated in healthcare settings, AI algorithms identify patterns, predict trends, and optimize various aspects of care delivery and staff workflows, leading to greater efficiency, improved resource utilization, and better patient outcomes.

AI algorithms can identify best practices and suggest evidence-based interventions tailored to individual patient needs. For example, AI can assist in identifying patients at high risk of complications or readmissions, allowing clinicians to intervene early and prevent adverse events. This proactive approach shortens length of stay, reduces hospital readmissions, and improves patient outcomes, all of which contribute to cost savings.

Moreover, AI optimizes care pathways by analyzing patient journeys across different care settings and identifying opportunities for improvement. By integrating data from EHRs, claims, and other sources, AI maps out the most effective and efficient pathways for managing specific conditions. This optimization helps reduce variations in care, improve resource utilization, and enhance patient satisfaction.

Hospitals and clinics must maintain adequate supplies of drugs, medical devices, and other essential materials to ensure uninterrupted patient care. AI can analyze usage patterns, predict future demand, and optimize ordering and stocking processes to reduce waste, minimize shortages, and control costs. By leveraging machine learning algorithms, AI also identifies opportunities for standardization and consolidation of supplies, leading to greater efficiency and cost savings. These improvements in supply chain management reduce operational expenses and free up resources for other critical areas of healthcare delivery.

Hospitals struggle with managing bed capacity, scheduling staff, and ensuring smooth patient transitions between different care settings. AI-powered tools can analyze historical and real-time data on patient admissions, discharges, and transfers to predict demand and optimize staff assignments and fixed asset utilization.

AI can generate optimized schedules that minimize wait times and maximize resource utilization by analyzing patient preferences, provider availability, and appointment durations. AI's advanced predictive analytics more accurately predict patient needs, allowing healthcare organizations to utilize fixed assets such as imaging equipment and surgical theaters more efficiently. In addition, AI predicts equipment failures, leading to proactive maintenance and repair to decrease downtime of revenue-generating equipment.

For example, AI systems can dynamically adjust staffing levels and resource allocation based on real-time patient flow and acuity data, leading to more efficient and responsive healthcare delivery. This dynamic optimization results in significant cost savings by ensuring the allocation of resources where they are needed most, reducing overstaffing in some areas while preventing understaffing in others.

AI-enhanced EHR systems improve patient referral processes and care coordination across healthcare settings. AI assists in identifying patients who require specialist care and matching them with the most appropriate and available providers based on specific patient needs.

Quality referrals require accurate and efficient communication of relevant patient information between primary care providers and specialists. AI-powered tools can automatically extract pertinent data from EHRs, such as medical history, diagnostic test results, and treatment plans, and generate comprehensive referral summaries. This automation reduces the administrative burden on healthcare providers and minimizes the risk of information gaps or errors during the referral process.

AI can assist in prioritizing referrals based on the urgency and complexity of patient needs. AI algorithms identify patients who require expedited referrals or additional support services by analyzing data from EHRs and other sources, including patient-reported outcomes and social determinants of health. This targeted approach ensures patients receive timely access to specialized care and improves overall health outcomes.

AI also optimizes the referral network by analyzing referral patterns and identifying opportunities for improvement. For example, AI tools can help identify areas where there may be a mismatch between the supply and demand of specialist services, enabling healthcare organizations to adjust their referral protocols or expand their provider networks accordingly. This data-driven approach leads to more efficient utilization of healthcare resources and reduces patient wait times.

RCM and Prior Authorization

Medicare's creation under President Lyndon Johnson in 1965 catalyzed a fundamental shift in healthcare documentation. The need for standardized medical procedure coding led to the American Medical Association to develop the Current Procedural Terminology (CPT) system in 1966. This first standardized medical coding system initially focused on surgical procedures and laid the foundation for modern healthcare reimbursement by providing a means to use a single code to document clinical work.

Medical coding is notoriously complex, requiring the error-prone translation of clinical documentation into standardized codes for billing purposes. NLP extracts relevant information from unstructured clinical notes more accurately than human coders and combine it with available structured data, improving coding accuracy. AI also assists coders by automating the analysis of clinical data and suggesting appropriate codes and modifiers. This automation reduces the likelihood of coding errors and improves the efficiency of the billing process.

Claims denials represent a major source of lost revenue for healthcare organizations. Estimates suggest that payers deny up to 20% of their first submissions of claims. This high denial rate incurs additional costs associated with appeals and resubmissions and impacts immediate cash flow.

AI algorithms can analyze historical claims data to identify patterns and risk factors associated with denials, such as missing documentation, incorrect coding, or lack of medical necessity. By flagging these issues proactively and allowing for documentation revision before submission, AI prevents denials before they occur.

By reducing the time and resources devoted to submitting and following up on authorization requests, providers can allocate their staff more efficiently to patient care activities and obtain timely reimbursements. In addition, faster authorization decisions reduce delays in care delivery, leading to better patient outcomes and lower overall healthcare costs.

By analyzing claims data in real time, AI prioritizes high-value claims and identifies those at risk of exceeding timely filing limits. This ensures that organizations submit claims promptly and accurately, reducing the risk of denials and reimbursement delays.

For insurers, AI-powered prior authorization systems can quickly analyze medical records, claims history, and clinical guidelines to make accurate and consistent authorization decisions. This automation reduces the need for manual review, decreasing processing times and administrative costs.

As AI continuously learns and improves, adapting to new clinical evidence and frequent policy changes, it helps ensure authorization decisions remain up-to-date and aligned with best practices and regulations. These RCM improvements depend upon robust interoperability so the provider and insurer can exchange complete medical record information.

Patients, too, can experience economic benefits from AI-enhanced prior authorization processes. With faster approvals, patients are less likely to delay receiving necessary treatments. This timely access to care leads to earlier interventions, preventing disease progression and reducing the need for more expensive treatments in the future. In addition, patients are less likely to obtain care not covered by their insurance, allowing them to seek alternative providers or adjust their treatment plans.

Machine learning models are becoming increasingly sophisticated in predicting patient propensity to pay, allowing healthcare organizations to tailor their collection strategies and improve overall revenue recovery. This targeted approach to collections enhances the efficiency of revenue recovery efforts, reducing bad debt and improving overall financial performance.

While AI offers excellent opportunities to improve RCM, organizations must ensure the accuracy and reliability of AI-powered solutions. Errors or inaccuracies have economic consequences for patients and healthcare organizations. As such, investment in rigorous testing, validation, and ongoing monitoring of AI tools is essential. While this represents an upfront cost, it delivers substantial long-term benefits.

Implementation Challenges

Cost: While the economic benefits of AI-enhanced EHR systems are considerable, it is important to consider the challenges and costs associated with their implementation. The initial investment required to upgrade existing EHR systems or implement new AI-powered platforms is substantial.

Additionally, the ongoing maintenance and updating of AI and ensuring compliance with evolving privacy and security regulations represent continuing costs that organizations balance against the savings and efficiency gains.

Models: If the data used to train AI models does not represent the targeted patient population or contains historical biases, the resulting algorithms may perpetuate or amplify these biases. These biases lead to disparities in care and worsen health outcomes for specific patient groups. Ensuring that AI algorithms use diverse and inclusive datasets regularly audited for fairness and equity is essential.

Cybersecurity: Healthcare data is highly sensitive, and using AI introduces new risks related to data breaches, unauthorized access, and misuse. Healthcare organizations should implement robust data governance frameworks and security measures to protect patient privacy and maintain trust in the healthcare system.

Change Management: Integrating AI into clinical workflows is disruptive and requires changes to existing processes and roles. Healthcare providers will need to adapt to new ways of interacting with EHR systems and interpreting AI-generated insights. This new workflow can lead to resistance to change and barriers to adoption. Overcoming these barriers requires clinicians' involvement in designing and implementing AI solutions and adequate training and support to ensure successful integration into clinical practice.

Technology: Automation bias, an overreliance on automated decision support, poses another risk to organizations and patients. While AI can provide valuable insights and recommendations, it is important to recognize that AI is not infallible and may not capture all relevant factors in a patient's care. Healthcare providers must maintain their critical thinking skills and use AI to support their clinical judgment rather than replace it.

Recent advancements in explainable AI (XAI) techniques have begun to address some of these challenges by making AI decision-making processes more transparent and interpretable.

As AI technologies mature, technology companies, startups, and investors are developing and commercializing new AI-powered healthcare solutions. There is significant investment and competition in healthcare AI, with established technology companies, startups, and healthcare organizations vying for market share. This competition is leading to the rapid development of new AI-powered products and services.

This rapid pace of technological change presents significant risks. AI healthcare technology must be safe, effective, and ethically sound. The rush to commercialize healthcare AI could lead to deploying poorly tested or validated systems, putting patients and organizations at risk.

Existing perverse incentives may create AI tools that degrade patient care. For instance, AI algorithms designed to optimize revenue generation without considering the appropriateness of care can lead to overutilization of services and increased healthcare costs. Therefore, AI solutions must prioritize patient well-being and clinical effectiveness over short-term financial gains.

There are concerns that AI's benefits may accrue disproportionately to wealthy and technologically advanced healthcare organizations, leaving smaller organizations and their underserved populations behind.

Stakeholders, including healthcare organizations, government regulatory bodies, and technology companies, should develop robust policies to prevent these problems and ensure that healthcare AI is focused on the best interests of patients and society. These policies include the creation of standards and regulations for creating and using AI in healthcare, as well as mechanisms for monitoring and mitigating harms. There must be a commitment to transparency, accountability, and ethical considerations.

Integrating healthcare AI requires balancing economic goals with patient care. To achieve the optimal balance, healthcare organizations should carefully consider the value proposition of AI adoption. Balance involves setting clear outcome metrics aligning with patient, provider, and societal interests. For example, AI tools that improve the accuracy of diagnoses, reduce medical errors, and enhance patient satisfaction can contribute to better clinical outcomes while driving financial benefits through reduced complications and readmissions.

While clinical documentation drives reimbursement, its most important use is in patient care. As healthcare organizations deploy AI tools for generating clinical summaries, they face critical questions about standards, validation, and risk management. My next *Bedside Consult* examines these challenges through the lens of AI-generated clinical summaries, offering insights into the careful balance between efficiency and clinical quality.

Bedside Consult: Navigating Risk—Standards Required for AI-Generated Clinical Summaries

The advent of AI in generating clinical summaries has presented unparalleled opportunities and significant challenges. As we stand on the cusp of integrating these technologies into everyday clinical practice, we must navigate these waters with caution and foresight.

The *JAMA* article, "AI-generated clinical summaries require more than accuracy," (Goodman, 2024) highlights the potential of large language models (LLMs) in streamlining information gathering from EHR systems. It underscores the necessity for transparently developing standards for LLM-generated clinical summaries and pragmatic clinical studies to ensure their safe and prudent deployment. This resonates deeply with my conviction that as we embrace AI in clinical settings, we must prioritize accuracy, transparency, and standards to mitigate misinformation risks.

AI-generated clinical summaries impact patient care and medical research. They promise to alleviate physician burnout and enhance clinical decision-making by providing succinct, relevant, and accurate summaries of complex patient data. However, without stringent standards and clear indications that these summaries are AI-generated, we risk introducing biases and inaccuracies into patient records—a scenario we must diligently avoid to ensure the highest patient care and safety standards.

Variability and Clinical Decision-Making

LLMs, by design, do not produce a single, definitive output for a given input. Instead, they generate summaries based on a complex interplay of factors, including their training data and the nuances of the algorithms that drive their predictions. This interplay means that even with identical prompts or clinical information, the summaries produced by LLMs can differ in detail, such as the conditions listed, the clinical history elements emphasized, or the organization and phrasing of the summary itself. Goodman's article illustrates this with examples where ChatGPT-4 prompts summarized deidentified clinical documents. This resulted in summaries that varied in the patient conditions listed and the clinical history elements emphasized.

Clinical Implications of Variability

This variability is not merely a technical issue; it has profound clinical implications. Organizing and framing information in a clinical summary influences clinician interpretations and subsequent decisions. Differences in summaries can nudge clinicians towards different diagnostic or treatment paths, intentionally or unintentionally, based on the information emphasized or omitted. This variability is particularly concerning given the high stakes in medical decision-making and the potential for such variability to impact patient care and outcomes. Also, any unreliable EHR data degrades its value in medical research.

To this end, standards development requires a focus on accuracy and includes measures to test for biases and errors that could have clinical implications. Such standards are the product of a collective effort involving not just technology developers but also clinicians, regulatory bodies, and other stakeholders in the healthcare ecosystem.

Furthermore, AI-generated summaries should be rigorously tested in clinical settings to quantify their benefits and risks before widespread adoption. While it is still unclear whether the responsibility for testing falls on the FDA, the technology companies developing these products, or the institutions implementing them, deploying *black box* LLMs without oversight is dangerous.

The probabilistic nature of LLMs presents a complex challenge for their application in generating clinical summaries. While these models hold the promise of streamlining the gathering of information from EHRs and improving the efficiency of clinical documentation, addressing the variability and uncertainty they introduce is crucial. Developing rigorous standards and conducting clinical studies to evaluate the impact of this variability on patient care are critical steps toward the safe and effective integration of AI technologies in healthcare.

Using artificial intelligence in healthcare operations represents a pivotal moment in the industry's evolution. While the economic benefits are compelling—from reduced administrative burden to streamlined operations and improved RCM—our ability to translate these efficiencies into better patient care and more equitable access to health services is the better measure of success. As healthcare organizations navigate this transformation, focusing on patient outcomes while leveraging AI's capabilities is crucial for ethically using AI in healthcare delivery.

CHAPTER II

Job Security and New Roles

In 1785, Edmund Cartwright invented the power loom, a machine that used water power to speed up the weaving process. Cartwright's power loom was a crucial step in the mechanization of textile manufacturing. Although it initially sparked fierce resistance from skilled weavers, by 1850, this mechanization created more textile jobs than ever before, albeit requiring different skills. The workers who adapted to operate the new machinery found themselves in higher-paying, less physically demanding roles, while those who resisted change struggled to maintain employment.

Integrating artificial intelligence (AI) into healthcare represents a transformative force, reshaping job roles and redefining job security. While disruptive, this shift heralds increased efficiency and innovation.

Strategizing how the workforce can adapt and flourish with healthcare AI requires a proactive approach. This approach should focus on continuous learning, interdisciplinary collaboration, and embracing AI's value as a tool for enhancement rather than replacement.

The journey through historical and technological transitions offers a rich tapestry of insights. While each transition is unique, these transitions share common themes of disruption, adaptation, and eventual integration, providing a valuable roadmap for how healthcare might navigate the shift to AI.

The Industrial Revolution stands out as a profound example. This era redefined employment and societal structures, shifting labor from manual to machine-assisted tasks. The initial disruption, marked by job displacement and societal upheaval, eventually led to unprecedented productivity, job creation, and improvements in the standard of living.

In healthcare, a similar pattern emerges with AI. Initial concerns over AI replacing jobs are giving way to a recognition of AI as a tool for advancing care delivery, improving patient outcomes, and enhancing clinician roles. The transition from manual to mechanized manufacturing during the Industrial Revolution parallels the current shift in healthcare from traditional methods to AI-assisted practices. AI is not replacing healthcare professionals but augmenting their roles, enabling them to provide more efficient and accurate care while reducing the burden of administrative work.

This historical example highlights a consistent pattern: technological advancements initially disrupt existing systems but ultimately lead to new opportunities. It emphasizes adaptability, continuous learning, and a proactive approach to embracing new technologies.

The pace of change with AI is significantly faster than previous technological revolutions. This rapid technological advancement signifies that the adaptation period may be shorter, requiring a more agile response from individuals and organizations.

Healthcare AI converts manual, repetitive tasks, such as clinical documentation coding, to more strategic, impactful work facilitated by AI's capability to process and analyze vast amounts of data efficiently. AI is also creating new roles.

Jobs such as AI healthcare analysts and AI ethics officers are becoming increasingly relevant. The AI healthcare analyst interprets data from AI systems to devise patient care strategies. At the same time, the AI ethics officer ensures that the AI implementation aligns with ethical, quality, and safety standards, addressing risks such as data privacy, algorithmic bias, and the impact on patient care.

While the rapid progression of healthcare AI brings groundbreaking advancements, it also challenges the status quo of healthcare jobs. These new roles and the modification of existing ones are happening at an unprecedented pace, often outstripping the ability of institutions to provide formal training programs.

Medical, nursing, and allied healthcare professions schools must incorporate AI and data science courses into their core curricula. There is a growing demand for interdisciplinary programs that combine healthcare, computer science, and ethics to produce professionals who can lead the responsible development and implementation of healthcare AI. Continuing education programs are crucial to help existing healthcare professionals adapt.

Healthcare organizations should proactively invest in training programs and continuous professional development to ensure their workforce can confidently utilize AI technologies. This training must extend beyond mere technical skills to include ethical decision-making, data privacy, and the impact on patient experience.

New Job Types

In 1894, Herman Hollerith revolutionized data management by inventing an electromechanical machine that used punch cards to record and summarize information. Originally developed to address the U.S. Census Bureau's inefficiencies, his machine dramatically reduced the time needed to complete a census from 7–8 years to just 2–3 years, showcasing the transformative power of automation. This innovation modernized data analysis and created an entirely new profession: *the data processing operator*. Hollerith later founded the company that would become International Business Machines (IBM), laying the groundwork for the information age and establishing foundational principles for modern computing and analytics.

The rapid advancement of AI has led to the creation of entirely new fields. For instance, computational medicine, which combines medical knowledge with AI and data science, is emerging as a crucial area of expertise. Similarly, the role of data scientists specializing in applying AI to healthcare data is becoming increasingly valuable.

AI also catalyzes the need for novel skill sets, such as the combination of data analytics proficiency, understanding of large language models, and the application of AI in clinical settings. This evolution necessitates a commitment to lifelong learning and professional development as healthcare workers try to adapt at the same pace as the introduction of new technologies.

Healthcare professionals must engage with data science, information technology, and ethics experts to better understand how AI tools work and their utility in healthcare. Organizations facilitate this by creating cross-functional teams and promoting knowledge-sharing platforms.

Lastly, it is essential to cultivate a mindset that views AI as a complementary asset for the workforce. Healthcare workers should see AI as a tool that enhances their capabilities and supports their decision-making processes, not as a threat to their roles. For example, AI-powered diagnostic tools can aid physicians in making more accurate diagnoses, but the physician's judgment remains irreplaceable. Healthcare leaders play a crucial role in fostering this mindset through clear communication about the role of AI, its benefits, and its impact on staff roles.

The transformation of medical roles through AI mirrors previous technological disruptions, offering valuable lessons for healthcare leaders. The evolution of office work presents a compelling parallel to healthcare's current transition. This historical example illustrates how workforce adaptation to new technologies can create unexpected opportunities for professional growth.

SideBar: From Typing Pools to Word Processing

The introduction of word processing technology in the 1970s and 1980s marks a pivotal transformation in office work. This transformation mainly affected typing pools, centralized departments where skilled typists traditionally handled all document creation and revision.

Before word processing, typing pools were essential components of most large organizations. These departments employed skilled typists who maintained high word-per-minute rates with accuracy. Speed and accuracy were crucial skills, as documents needing multiple revisions required complete retyping. Typing pool workers typically had limited career advancement opportunities and were often viewed as support staff rather than knowledge workers.

The introduction of word processing systems fundamentally changed document creation and management. These new systems revolutionized office work by offering unprecedented document editing capabilities without complete retyping. The technology brought sophisticated formatting options that were impossible with traditional typewriters. Most importantly, word processing introduced the ability to store and retrieve documents electronically, fundamentally changing how offices manage their information. Including features such as search and replace dramatically improved productivity, while the ability to standardize document formats brought new consistency to organizational documentation.

The transition period revealed two distinct groups within the typing pools. The first group consisted of adaptive workers who embraced the new technology, learning word processing skills while leveraging their typing proficiency. The second group comprised workers who resisted the change and focused solely on traditional typing skills.

Those who adapted to word processing experienced significant career benefits. Their embrace of new technology resulted in higher salaries reflecting their enhanced technical skills. These workers found their job responsibilities expanding beyond mere typing, opening new career paths in information management and document processing. Many transitioned into various departments rather than remaining in centralized pools, and some advanced into supervisory or training roles.

In contrast, those who did not adapt faced increasingly difficult career prospects. Their job opportunities gradually diminished, and their wages decreased. As word processing became ubiquitous across industries, many workers eventually faced job displacement.

The transition to word processing created fundamental changes in office dynamics. Once centralized in typing pools, document creation became distributed across departments as more workers gained access to word-processing technology. Typing skills evolved from a specialized profession to become part of the general office competency requirements. New roles emerged, focusing on technology training and support, while the emphasis shifted from specialized typing skills to broader computer literacy.

This transformation is a model for future technological transitions in the workplace. It demonstrates that adaptability and willingness to learn new skills are crucial for career longevity. Workers discover that technical proficiency could lead to career advancement, while traditional specialized skills must evolve with technological changes. The experience shows how workplace roles are fundamentally reshaped by technology.

The transition from typing pools to word processing represents a classic case of technological disruption in the workplace. Those who adapted their skills survived the transition and often thrived, while those who resisted change faced career difficulties. The transformation highlights how technological advancement creates new career pathways and opportunities for workers willing to embrace change and develop new skills. This pattern would repeat itself in subsequent decades with other technological advances, making this case study particularly relevant for understanding workplace adaptation to technological change.

As organizations face technological disruption, the lessons learned from this transition remain relevant, demonstrating the importance of adaptability and continuous learning in maintaining career growth and job security.

Economics of Workforce Transformation

In 1956, Leonard Skeggs revolutionized laboratory diagnostics by developing the first fully automated system capable of measuring glucose, urea, and calcium levels in blood samples. This invention addressed the growing demand for faster, more accurate, and scalable medical testing. Shortly after, Skeggs' innovation was commercialized by Technicon as the *AutoAnalyzer*, a groundbreaking machine that performed blood analysis with minimal manual intervention. The AutoAnalyzer dramatically improved efficiency, reduced human error, and standardized test results by automating complex chemical analyses. This milestone marked the beginning of modern clinical chemistry automation, paving the way for the high-throughput laboratory systems that underpin today's healthcare diagnostics.

If properly implemented, AI can drive significant economic efficiency. AI-driven diagnostic tools and predictive analytics reduce operational costs by enhancing accuracy and reducing ineffective or unnecessary tests and treatments. This efficiency translates to direct cost savings for healthcare providers and directly benefits patients through quicker, more accurate diagnoses and treatment plans.

This efficiency directly impacts job security. As AI automates routine tasks, especially in administrative and data management areas, there is a realistic concern that AI-powered automation will displace jobs traditionally performed by humans. It is crucial to address these concerns proactively by identifying areas where the workforce can be retrained or upskilled. For example, organizations can retrain administrative staff for AI system oversight, data analysis, or patient engagement roles that are augmented, not replaced, by AI.

AI's ability to streamline operations and provide innovative diagnostic and treatment solutions opens new avenues for service expansion and business development. This growth is not limited to healthcare providers but extends to tech companies, life science firms, and other stakeholders involved in the broader healthcare marketplace. The economic ripple effect of AI will lead to the creation of entirely new industries and jobs focused on digital health solutions and alternative patient care models.

While the long-term economic benefits are significant, the short-term costs of AI implementation, including technology acquisition, workforce training, and system integration, will be financially challenging for many healthcare organizations. This economic dis-parity may lead to a digital divide, where only well-resourced orga-nizations can fully leverage AI technologies, leaving those other institutions and workers at a strategic disadvantage.

Integrating AI with emerging technologies like robotics, nano-technology, and genetic engineering will open new healthcare fields. This convergence of technologies will create roles that we can hardly imagine today, much like how the smartphone revolution created new job categories that did not exist a decade ago.

As AI systems expand their capabilities, there will be a growing emphasis on the uniquely human aspects of healthcare. Empathy, complex ethical decision-making, and the ability to handle ambigu-ous situations are areas where human healthcare professionals con-tinue to excel. Future healthcare roles will increasingly emphasize these human qualities, with AI handling more of care's mundane and routine aspects.

Managing this unprecedented technological transformation requires new organizational leadership that did not exist a decade ago. The healthcare industry has historically created new executive positions to manage transformative changes, as evidenced by the emergence of the Chief Medical Information Officer (CMIO) role during the electronic health record (EHR) system implementation period. As explained in my next *Bedside Consult*, today's AI revo-lution similarly demands specialized executive oversight to ensure successful integration while focusing on clinical outcomes.

Bedside Consult: Why Every Organization Needs a CAIO

As AI rapidly transforms industries and reshapes organizations' operations, the need for dedicated leadership to navigate this complex landscape is increasingly apparent. Just as the introduction of EHRs necessitated the creation of the CMIO role, the rise of AI calls for a new executive position: the Chief Artificial Intelligence Officer (CAIO).

The CAIO is a critical link between an organization's technology, operations, and strategic vision. This role ensures that AI initiatives align with the organization's goals and operational realities, bridging the gap between technical capabilities and business needs. By providing focused expertise and oversight, the CAIO guides the organization through the intricacies of AI deployment, from data ethics and governance to integration with existing systems.

The CAIO's role is particularly crucial in healthcare. AI can revolutionize patient care, modernize operations, and enhance medical research. However, implementing AI in healthcare presents unique challenges, such as ensuring patient privacy, maintaining data security, and navigating complex regulatory requirements. A healthcare CAIO requires a deep understanding of the medical field and AI technologies to address these challenges and drive AI adoption effectively.

Senior Level Appointment

Appointing a CAIO at the senior level brings numerous benefits to an organization. By having a dedicated executive overseeing AI initiatives, organizations ensure that AI strategies align with overall business goals and are implemented efficiently. The CAIO drives innovation and competitive advantage by identifying opportunities for AI to enhance products, services, and internal processes, keeping the organization at the forefront of technological advancements.

Moreover, the CAIO provides the necessary leadership to navigate the complex ethical and regulatory landscape surrounding AI. As AI systems become more sophisticated and ubiquitous, concerns around data privacy, algorithmic bias, and transparency will only intensify. The CAIO can develop robust governance frameworks and ensure compliance with emerging regulations, mitigating legal and reputational risks.

To effectively fulfill their role, the CAIO requires a dedicated staff to develop, implement, and test AI tools. This team consists of data scientists, AI engineers, and domain experts collaborating to create AI solutions tailored to the organization's specific needs. By having an in-house AI development team, organizations maintain control over their AI assets, ensure the security of sensitive data, and adapt quickly to changing requirements. In addition, the team can evaluate vendor products for efficacy and safety.

Organizations should model the structure of the CAIO's office after the office of the CMIO or Chief Operating Officer (COO). Just as the CMIO manages technology initiatives and the COO oversees operations, the CAIO should have the authority and resources to manage AI projects from conception to deployment. Their authority includes setting priorities, allocating budgets, and measuring the impact of AI interventions on key performance indicators.

To ensure that AI is integrated seamlessly across the organization, the CAIO or a senior staff member is included in committees run by other senior executives. In healthcare, this means having a seat in discussions about clinical care, patient experience, operations, and information technology. By actively participating in these committees, the CAIO can provide valuable insights into leveraging AI to improve outcomes, streamline processes, and enhance decision-making.

Rare Combination of Skills

The ideal candidate for a healthcare CAIO should possess a rare combination of qualifications. A medical degree is essential to understand the nuances of patient care and the clinical decision-making process. A deep understanding of healthcare IT systems is necessary to integrate AI solutions with existing infrastructure effectively. Experience in patient quality and safety initiatives ensures that AI applications prioritize patient well-being and adhere to stringent safety standards. Finally, a strong background in analytics is essential to harness the power of data-driven insights and optimize AI performance.

As healthcare organizations increasingly rely on AI to improve patient outcomes and operations, and drive research breakthroughs, the role of the CAIO will only grow in importance. By appointing a dedicated executive to lead AI initiatives, organizations will be well-positioned to capitalize on this technology's transformative potential while navigating its complexities and challenges.

In conclusion, the rise of AI demands a new type of leadership in every organization, particularly in healthcare. With their unique medical expertise, technological acumen, and strategic vision, the CAIO is best suited to guide organizations through the AI revolution. By prioritizing the appointment of a CAIO, organizations can unlock the full capabilities of AI while ensuring its responsible and ethical use. As we move into an increasingly AI-driven future, the CAIO will undoubtedly become an indispensable executive team member, driving innovation, efficiency, and improved outcomes across the board.

The transformation of healthcare roles through artificial intelligence represents both a challenge and an opportunity for the healthcare workforce. Just as the Industrial Revolution, the computing era, and the adoption of EHRs reshaped professional roles, AI catalyzes the evolution of healthcare careers. However, this transformation differs in its unprecedented pace and scope. Success requires healthcare organizations to balance technological advancement with human expertise, ensuring AI is a tool for enhancement rather than replacement. Organizations that invest in workforce development, create clear career advancement pathways, and maintain focus on the uniquely human aspects of healthcare will thrive in this AI-enhanced future. The key lies in embracing change and using AI to improve patient care and professional satisfaction. As healthcare continues its AI journey, our industry must remember that technology, no matter how advanced, serves to augment rather than replace the human judgment, empathy, and ethical decision-making that form the cornerstone of quality healthcare delivery.

CHAPTER 12

Patient Privacy and Cybersecurity

In 1928, Justice Louis Brandeis established a foundational principle for American privacy law in his dissent in Olmstead v. United States, describing privacy as *the right to be let alone.* This right, he argued, was among the most comprehensive of rights and the most valued by civilized people. Nearly a century later, Brandeis's prescient concern for privacy takes on new urgency. While he worried about telephone wiretaps, today's healthcare privacy challenges involve vast datasets of protected health information (PHI) used to train artificial intelligence (AI) systems, introducing unprecedented risks to patient privacy that Brandeis could never have imagined.

The centralization of large PHI datasets for healthcare AI model training creates high-value targets for cybercriminals, who recognize the monetary value of this sensitive information. Even with robust de-identification measures in place, the complexity of healthcare data makes it possible to re-identify individuals through sophisticated pattern analysis and cross-referencing techniques. This risk is particularly acute as these datasets often contain detailed medical histories, genetic information, and personal insurance and financial information. Privacy breaches have far-reaching consequences beyond immediate financial and reputational damage to people and organizations.

Compromised PHI affects patients' insurability, employment opportunities, and personal relationships. Release of health information sometimes leads to discrimination or social stigma. For healthcare organizations, privacy breaches can result in severe regulatory penalties, loss of patient trust, and long-term damage to their ability to deliver effective care.

At the heart of healthcare AI lies a paradox: developing accurate, reliable AI models demands vast amounts of detailed patient data, yet each additional piece of information in the training set exponentially increases privacy risks. This paradox creates a complex balance between model performance and patient privacy protection.

Modern machine learning (ML) models, especially deep learning systems, demonstrate a near-insatiable appetite for data. A typical medical imaging AI model might require millions of labeled images for clinical-grade accuracy. Natural language processing models used for clinical documentation need extensive training on patient records to understand medical terminology and context.

Collecting and storing PHI for AI training introduces multiple points of vulnerability. Healthcare organizations must navigate complex data-sharing agreements, secure data transfer mechanisms, and maintain appropriate access controls across numerous systems and stakeholders. Organizations compound the problem by aggregating data from multiple sources to create a single, comprehensive training dataset.

Unlike traditional medical records, which typically reside within well-defined system boundaries, AI training data require access by development teams, data scientists, and training infrastructure. Maintaining clear lineage and appropriate security controls becomes increasingly complex as data moves through various systems and processes. Organizations must ensure Health Insurance Portability and Accountability Act (HIPAA) compliance across distributed storage systems and cloud platforms used for AI training, often spanning multiple vendors and geographic locations. Expanded access creates new opportunities for unauthorized access or data leakage.

Data Collection and Storage Vulnerabilities

Before developers use PHI for model training, it typically undergoes extensive preprocessing to prepare it for ML. This critical phase introduces several privacy vulnerabilities:

Data Normalization: Standardizing data formats and values can inadvertently expose sensitive information through logging or temporary files. For example, when normalizing dates of birth to a standard format, intermediate files might contain unencrypted patient identifiers alongside medical information.

Feature Engineering: Creating meaningful features for the training of AI models often requires combining different aspects of the raw data from patient records. Unique combinations of characteristics could make it easier to re-identify individuals. Even when individual data elements are appropriately de-identified, the relationships between features can create unique fingerprints that enable re-identification.

Data Augmentation: Techniques used to expand training datasets, such as generating synthetic variations of medical images or patient records, can inadvertently encode personal information in difficult-to-detect and control ways.

Training AI models introduces additional privacy risks that many organizations overlook. One such risk is the *AI memorization risk,* where modern deep learning models demonstrated an alarming capability to memorize specific examples from their training data. Memorization means that the model remembers and reproduces verbatim snippets of training text or reconstructs detailed features of training images, which could lead to privacy violations.

This memorization risk is concerning, as even small fragments of remembered information could constitute HIPAA violations. For example, a large language model (LLM) trained on clinical notes might inadvertently encode and later reproduce specific patient diagnoses or treatment details. Similarly, imaging models might retain unique identifying features from radiological scans or pathology slides.

The distributed nature of modern AI training infrastructure compounds these risks. Training occurs across multiple graphics processing unit clusters in different physical locations or cloud environments. Each additional node in the training infrastructure represents a point of vulnerability where PHI might be exposed, adding to the complexity of ensuring data security.

Model Deployment and Production Risks

In 1969, the U.S. Department of Defense released the Advance Research Projects Agency Network (ARPANET), the first system connecting computers and the internet's precursor. Early efforts focused on simple access controls and encryption, a far cry from the sophisticated protections needed for modern AI systems. Yet those pioneering security efforts established principles that still guide our approach to protecting sensitive data in distributed systems.

The deployment phase of AI systems introduces new challenges encompassing far more than traditional healthcare information technology rollouts. When organizations deploy AI models into production environments, they access live patient data, creating dynamic privacy risks that evolve each time they access patient data.

Production AI systems typically require complex infrastructure that spans multiple environments and security domains. A typical deployment might include:

Edge Computing Nodes: Models deployed directly on medical devices or clinical settings must process patient data in real time while maintaining HIPAA compliance. These edge deployments often operate in environments with varying physical and network security levels, creating unique challenges for protecting the model and the data it processes.

API Endpoints: Healthcare organizations use Application Programming Interfaces (APIs) to integrate AI models with clinical systems. These endpoints must be carefully secured to prevent unauthorized access while maintaining accessibility for legitimate users. Recent security incidents have demonstrated that cybercriminals can exploit inadequately protected API endpoints using carefully crafted queries to extract sensitive patient information.

Cloud Infrastructure: Many healthcare AI systems rely on cloud computing resources for scalability and performance. This reliance introduces additional complexity in ensuring HIPAA compliance across distributed systems, mainly when dealing with multi-cloud or hybrid deployments. Organizations should maintain transparent data governance and security controls across all environments where PHI is processed or stored.

Security, Privacy, and Threats

How AI systems operate presents unique privacy challenges that require sophisticated protection mechanisms:

Model Inference Protection: When AI models process live patient data, each inference operation creates a point of data exposure. Cybersecure organizations implement robust monitoring systems to detect and prevent unauthorized access or attempts to extract sensitive information through model interactions.

Access Control and Authentication: Healthcare AI systems often require different access levels for various user roles, from clinical staff to researchers and administrators. Implementing granular access controls while maintaining usability demands sophisticated identity and access management systems that adapt to changing organizational needs.

Audit Trail Management: HIPAA compliance requires maintaining detailed audit trails of all PHI access and usage. This requirement extends to tracking model interactions, training data usage, and system modifications of AI systems. Organizations must implement comprehensive logging and monitoring systems while ensuring the audit trails do not become vectors for privacy breaches.

Recent advances in privacy-preserving ML offer promising solutions for protecting PHI while maintaining AI system effectiveness:

Federated Learning Implementation: This distributed learning approach trains models across multiple healthcare organizations without centralizing patient data. Recent implementations have successfully trained AI models across institutions while maintaining strict data privacy. However, organizations must consider federated learning systems' computational overhead and coordination effort.

Differential Privacy Advances: New techniques for implementing differential privacy provide mathematical guarantees about privacy preservation while minimizing the impact on model performance. Recent research has shown effective approaches for balancing privacy budgets with model utility in clinical applications.

Homomorphic Encryption Applications: The maturation of homomorphic encryption technologies enables the computation of encrypted patient data without exposure. While computational overhead remains challenging, recent optimizations make these techniques increasingly practical for specific healthcare applications.

Secure Enclaves: These enclaves provide hardware-level isolation for sensitive computations, though IT staff must carefully consider implementation complexities and performance overhead when choosing this approach.

The threat to healthcare AI systems continues to expand:

Model Extraction Attacks: Sophisticated adversaries can reconstruct training data from deployed AI models by carefully analyzing model outputs. These attacks are increasingly efficient, requiring fewer queries to extract sensitive information.

Transfer Learning Vulnerabilities: The common practice of using pre-trained models introduces privacy leakage from the original training data. Recent research shows that models can retain and expose sensitive information even after using new datasets for fine-tuning.

Supply Chain Attacks: The complex ecosystem of AI development tools creates opportunities for malicious actors to compromise systems by targeting a single node. Cybersecure organizations implement robust supply-chain technology security measures to guard against these threats.

As organizations grapple with these evolving threats, differential privacy is a powerful tool. It provides rigorous guarantees for privacy protection that seemed impossible just a decade ago.

Side Bar: Differential Privacy Techniques

Differential privacy represents one of the most significant advances in protecting patient privacy in healthcare AI systems. At its core, this mathematical framework provides a way to measure and control the privacy risk when using patient data in AI model training and deployment. Unlike traditional anonymization techniques that remove obvious identifiers, differential privacy offers provable guarantees about the level of privacy protection provided.

Consider a healthcare organization training an AI model to predict patient readmission risks. Without differential privacy, the model might inadvertently memorize specific details about individual patients, making it possible for attackers to extract this information by carefully analyzing the model's outputs. Differential privacy prevents this by adding carefully calibrated random noise to the data during training. Data scientists can precisely control the amount of noise to maintain the overall statistical usefulness of the data while making it mathematically impossible to determine whether or not any specific patient's information was used in training.

Implementing differential privacy requires organizations to work within a privacy budget. This budget quantifies how much information about individual patients can be revealed through interactions with the AI system. The system consumes some of this budget whenever it processes data or responds to queries. When the budget is exhausted, the system stops processing data to maintain its privacy guarantees. The budget is reset periodically based on the organization's needs and the demands of the AI tool.

Major healthcare systems now use differential privacy training methods for developing diagnostic models across multiple institutions. This approach allows organizations to build more accurate models using data from various sources while maintaining strict privacy controls.

However, implementing differential privacy requires careful consideration of tradeoffs between privacy protection and model usefulness. Adding too much random noise can make models less accurate, while adding too little might not provide adequate privacy protection. Organizations must carefully calibrate these parameters based on the sensitivity of the data and specific use cases. For instance, genetic data typically requires more robust privacy parameters than general demographic information due to its uniquely identifying nature.

Researchers demonstrated the effectiveness of differential privacy through rigorous mathematical proofs and practical implementations. The National Institute of Standards and Technology (NIST) now recommends differential privacy as a critical component of privacy-preserving ML in healthcare, particularly for applications involving sensitive patient information. Recent studies have shown that properly implemented differential privacy prevents even sophisticated model inversion attacks while maintaining clinical utility.

Organizations implementing differential privacy should also consider the operational implications of privacy budget management. This includes developing clear policies for budget allocation across different applications, monitoring budget consumption, and establishing procedures for when privacy budgets are exhausted.

Differential privacy continues to evolve as researchers develop more sophisticated implementations tailored to healthcare applications. Recent advances include dynamic privacy budget allocation methods based on data sensitivity and improved techniques for maintaining model utility under strict privacy constraints. These developments make differential privacy an increasingly practical tool for protecting patient privacy in AI systems.

♒

The emergence of industry-specific security standards for healthcare AI is creating new compliance challenges. These standards often require continuous monitoring and validation of privacy controls, moving beyond periodic assessments to real-time compliance verification. Organizations must implement automated systems that track compliance across multiple frameworks while adapting to new requirements as they emerge.

Cross-border data protection rules are increasingly complex for healthcare AI systems operating internationally. Dynamic compliance validation systems allow organizations to adjust privacy controls based on the specific requirements of different jurisdictions. These systems maintain comprehensive audit trails demonstrating compliance while enabling the efficient operation of global initiatives.

Recommendations for Healthcare Organizations

In 1943, Alan Turing, a WWII cryptographer at Britain's Bletchley Park, revolutionized cryptography while working to break the *German Enigma* code. His team discovered how seemingly innocuous patterns in encrypted messages could reveal sensitive information, directly paralleling modern concerns about information leakage from AI models. Turing demonstrated how mathematical techniques could protect sensitive information while enabling critical analysis—a principle underlying modern privacy-preserving AI techniques like homomorphic encryption. The British Government kept Turing's groundbreaking work classified until the 1970s, including his *Banburismus* process, which used probability and statistics for cryptanalysis—a remarkable precursor to modern privacy-preserving ML methods.

Healthcare organizations implementing AI systems must adopt a comprehensive approach to protecting PHI. This protection requires careful attention to technical and organizational measures and a thorough evaluation of vendors and partners. Recent privacy breaches demonstrate that vendor selection requires a sophisticated evaluation process that goes far beyond traditional security assessments.

Healthcare organizations begin vendor evaluation by examining technical capabilities to protect PHI. This assessment starts with understanding how vendors architect their systems. Leading vendors implement sophisticated end-to-end encryption using current NIST-approved algorithms; however, the implementation details are critically important.

Vendor evaluations begin with a thorough review of security certifications, including SOC 2 Type II reports and HITRUST certifications. However, certifications alone are insufficient. Thorough evaluation requires organizations to assess a vendor's data handling practices, security controls, and incident response capabilities. This evaluation should carefully review model development and training practices, mainly how the models protect PHI throughout these processes.

When examining vendor architectures, organizations scrutinize data segregation protocols. Modern healthcare AI systems often process data from multiple organizations, making isolation between environments crucial. Responsible vendors implement sophisticated multi-tenant architectures that prevent data leakage between clients. These systems typically employ dedicated encryption keys for each organization, managed through Hardware

Security Modules (HSMs) that provide additional protection for cryptographic operations.

The handling of PHI during model training requires scrutiny. Responsible vendors now implement privacy-preserving ML techniques such as differential privacy or federated learning. However, the mere presence of these technologies does not guarantee adequate protection. Organizations must understand how vendors implement these techniques, including their approach to privacy budgets and how they enforce these budgets during model development.

A vendor's approach to incident response and breach management deserves attention, as AI-related privacy breaches often require specialized detection and response capabilities. Responsible vendors implement automated detection systems to identify privacy leaks, including model inversion attempts and unauthorized access patterns. They maintain clear procedures for containing AI-related privacy incidents and can demonstrate regular testing of these procedures through documented demonstrations.

Contractual protections are crucial in vendor relationships, mainly through Business Associate Agreements (BAAs) that specifically address AI systems. These agreements go beyond standard BAA language to include requirements that directly address privacy protection in AI systems. Organizations must require vendors to implement detailed encryption standards, maintain minimum technical controls for PHI protection, and conduct regular privacy impact assessments. The agreements require clearly defined breach notification timelines and establish liability allocation for failing to protect PHI.

Once an organization establishes a vendor relationship, ongoing monitoring becomes essential. Healthcare organizations should implement continuous monitoring processes focusing on privacy impact metrics and regular evaluation of model behavior for leakage of PHI. This monitoring includes periodic vendor security assessments, penetration test results, and a review of privacy incident history. Cybersecure organizations also establish transparent processes for evaluating vendor implementations of system enhancements and updates to their privacy protection processes.

Recent guidance from the Office for Civil Rights in the U.S. Department of Health and Human Services emphasizes the importance of vendor selection in maintaining HIPAA compliance for AI systems. NIST also published detailed frameworks for evaluating healthcare AI vendors, providing organizations with structured approaches to vendor assessment. These resources and lessons learned from recent privacy breaches give healthcare organizations the tools to make informed vendor selection decisions.

As healthcare AI evolves, organizations should change their vendor evaluation processes to ensure rigorous assessment of vendor privacy protection capabilities. Recent breaches demonstrate that the cost of inadequate vendor evaluation is severe. Still, organizations implementing thorough detailed evaluation processes can reduce their risk of privacy incidents while advancing their AI initiatives.

Recent events demonstrate the importance of technical solutions and organizational controls that form the foundation of AI security. My next *Bedside Consult* examines how cybersecurity threats could derail the progress of AI-driven healthcare, offering practical insights for healthcare leaders navigating these challenges.

Bedside Consult: Will Hackers Derail AI-Driven Healthcare?

AI and LLMs are revolutionizing healthcare, offering unprecedented opportunities to enhance patient care, streamline operations, and drive innovation. However, as we embrace these transformative technologies, we must confront a sobering reality: AI systems are vulnerable to malicious attacks. This susceptibility poses significant risks to patient safety, data integrity, and the financial stability of healthcare organizations.

The Current Landscape: Cybersecurity Challenges

Recent events have underscored the urgency of addressing cybersecurity in healthcare. Numerous healthcare providers have fallen victim to ransomware attacks, compromising large patient datasets critical for care delivery. The high-profile hack of United-Health Group's Change Healthcare, which led to substantial delays in provider payments and a non-verified ransom payout of $22 million with overall costs exceeding $1 billion, is a stark reminder of the sector's vulnerability. These incidents highlight a troubling truth: if traditional healthcare IT systems are susceptible to such attacks, AI systems—with their complex architectures and often opaque decision-making processes—may be even more vulnerable.

The Unique Vulnerabilities of AI Systems

The AI Safety Institute in the United Kingdom recently published a groundbreaking report revealing that every major LLM can be *jailbroken* or compromised. This alarming finding underscores a fundamental challenge in AI security: unlike traditional software, AI systems are not written line by line with code. Instead, they are more akin to vast arrays of numbers that can perform remarkable tasks, but their inner workings are often obscure even to their creators.

This opacity makes patching vulnerabilities in AI systems exceptionally difficult. As one expert in the field noted, "A lot of the stuff that we do for cybersecurity and safety simply does not apply to AI systems in the same way as other forms of software." When a vulnerability is discovered in traditional software, programmers can examine the code, fix the problem, and deploy a patch. With AI systems, this straightforward approach is often impossible.

The Stakes: Consequences of Compromised AI

The consequences of compromised AI are profound. Hackers could manipulate AI models to produce inaccurate diagnoses, recommend inappropriate treatments, or generate fraudulent insurance claims. Since healthcare constitutes over 18% of the United States GDP, the financial incentives for bad actors to exploit these systems are substantial. Moreover, the inherent complexity of AI models, coupled with the difficulty in examining their training data and decision-making processes, compounds the challenge of detecting and mitigating such breaches.

The threat extends beyond direct patient care. AI systems are increasingly integrated into critical infrastructure, including healthcare facilities. If these systems are compromised, the consequences could be catastrophic, disrupting essential services and risking lives.

The Challenge of Distinguishing Reality from Fabrication

Another concern of healthcare AI is generating persuasive false information. As Jack Dorsey, former CEO of Twitter, warned, within the next five to ten years, it may become nearly impossible to differentiate between real and AI-generated content. "The only truth you have is what you can verify yourself with your experience," said Dorsey. He advised corporate leaders to verify everything as technology increasingly blurs the lines between real and fake. The prospect of being unable to trust AI tools presents significant challenges for healthcare professionals who rely on accurate information for decision-making and patient care.

Strategies for Securing AI in Healthcare

To address these challenges, healthcare leaders must take proactive steps:

Adoption of Best Practices*:* Implementing robust cybersecurity measures is non-negotiable, including regular vulnerability testing by providers, payers, and AI developers.

Continuous Evaluation: LLMs require continual assessment for accuracy and value and detailed documentation of model training and testing procedures.

Transparency and Accountability: Healthcare executives should demand transparency in AI development and security measures. This transparency extends to prompt notification of any security breaches, like the requirements for unauthorized releases of protected health information under HIPAA.

Regulatory Framework: There is a pressing need for regulations that hold AI developers accountable for the security of their tools. This framework includes penalties for inadequate security measures and mandates disclosure of steps taken to prevent hacking.

Industry-Wide Standards: Healthcare leaders must push for comprehensive standards in AI development and deployment, emphasizing performance, security, and ethical considerations.

Pilot Approaches: Organizations should consider starting with pilot projects using synthetic or anonymized data to test AI systems before full-scale implementation.

The Path Forward: Collaboration and Vigilance

As a physician dedicated to leveraging information technology to enhance patient care, I cannot overstate the importance of addressing these challenges. The potential of AI in healthcare is immense, but so are the risks if we fail to secure these systems adequately.

The path forward requires collaboration between healthcare providers, AI developers, policymakers, and cybersecurity experts. Only through such concerted efforts can we ensure that AI remains a force for good in healthcare, delivering on its promise to improve patient outcomes and operational efficiency without compromising security or ethical standards.

Balancing Innovation and Security

As this new AI era in healthcare emerges, let us embrace AI's opportunity while remaining clear-eyed about the challenges to overcome and realize its full potential. By demanding transparency, implementing robust security measures, and fostering a culture of continuous vigilance, we can harness the power of AI while safeguarding the integrity of our healthcare systems.

The future of healthcare lies in our ability to innovate responsibly, balancing AI's transformative power with the paramount need to protect patient safety and data integrity. As healthcare leaders, we must navigate this complex landscape, ensuring that AI's promise in healthcare is fulfilled without compromising the trust and well-being of those we serve.

The evolution of privacy protection mirrors the broader history of technological advancement. From Brandeis's *right to be let alone* to today's sophisticated differential privacy algorithms, each era has demanded new approaches to protecting patient information.

Success requires balancing technical innovation with ethical obligations, regulatory compliance with operational efficiency, and, most importantly, the promise of AI-driven healthcare with the fundamental right to privacy. Those who master this balance will define the future of healthcare delivery, creating systems that earn and maintain patient trust while harnessing AI's transformative potential to improve care delivery and clinical outcomes.

Success requires more than simply implementing current best practices—organizations must develop flexible, forward-looking approaches that adapt to emerging threats and evolving regulatory requirements. The future of healthcare AI depends on maintaining patient trust through a demonstrable commitment to privacy protection, requiring ongoing investment in advanced technologies and sophisticated controls.

PART III

Leading Tomorrow's Healthcare: AI Transformation

In Parts I and II, we explored the fundamental concepts and advanced applications of healthcare artificial intelligence (AI). Now, we turn to the most critical challenge: successful implementation. Let me be direct—technical sophistication alone will not guarantee success in healthcare AI initiatives. Even the most advanced AI systems fail without effective change management, trust building, and alignment with organizational goals. The pages ahead provide a practical roadmap for navigating these challenges while ensuring AI serves its ultimate purpose: improving patient care.

We begin by examining the delicate balance between AI's benefits and risks in healthcare settings. We review a comprehensive framework for evaluating and managing clinical and operational risks, with specific strategies for maximizing AI's benefits while maintaining the highest patient safety and care quality standards. From continuous testing and validation protocols to performance monitoring, we explore essential approaches that ensure AI systems enhance rather than compromise care delivery. Most importantly, we will understand the importance of establishing robust frameworks for evaluating AI systems before implementation and developing comprehensive validation studies that assess performance across diverse patient populations and clinical scenarios.

Implementation demands careful attention to alignment between AI capabilities and healthcare needs. I guide you through the principles for designing and deploying AI systems that serve patients and address societal needs. We learn how to embed ethical, transparent, and rights-focused principles into AI strategies while ensuring patient privacy and safety remain paramount. Success requires establishing comprehensive standards for AI development and implementation, including clear protocols for human oversight that ensure AI augments rather than replaces clinical judgment.

Trust emerges as a central challenge in healthcare AI implementation. We confront the reality of AI *hallucinations* and their impact on patient care, examining why these AI-generated errors occur and how to prevent them from affecting clinical decisions. We review concrete strategies for building and maintaining trust among healthcare professionals, patients, and stakeholders. Most crucially, we will learn approaches to *algorithmovigilance*—the continuous monitoring and analysis of AI systems—and how to implement *AI safety nets* that catch errors before they impact patient care.

The transformation demands building effective teams and managing organizational change. I provide strategies to create and lead interdisciplinary teams that bridge the gap between clinical excellence and technological innovation. We review frameworks for effective collaboration, including structured communication protocols and regular cross-functional reviews. We explore the art of prompt engineering—crafting inputs that train AI systems to produce desired responses—and learn how to bring together clinical specialists, prompt engineers, data scientists, AI ethicists, and healthcare informaticists in ways that maximize each role's contribution.

Finally, we examine workforce transformation, the crucial element for long-term success. We will learn comprehensive approaches to managing the human aspects of change effectively, with strategies for engaging stakeholders at all levels, from frontline clinicians to administrative staff. Success requires creating effective training programs, establishing feedback mechanisms, and demonstrating genuine commitment to incorporating staff input into implementation decisions. We review the importance of professional development, which helps staff learn new skills in data interpretation, AI-assisted decision-making, and workflow optimization.

Throughout Part III, I emphasize practical, actionable insights you can apply in your organization. The challenges we explore are not theoretical; they represent the real-world obstacles we must overcome to implement AI technologies successfully. You will gain frameworks, strategies, and specific tools needed to navigate these challenges effectively while avoiding common pitfalls that can derail AI initiatives.

Successful AI implementation requires a holistic approach that considers technology's impact on people, processes, and organizational culture. We must balance technological sophistication with human factors—engaging stakeholders, building sustainable processes, and maintaining an unwavering focus on patient care. Building on the foundational knowledge established in Parts 1 and 2, these pages will help you develop comprehensive strategies for implementing AI to enhance rather than disrupt healthcare delivery.

The transformation of healthcare through artificial intelligence is not about adopting new technologies—it is about reimagining how we deliver care to benefit patients and society. Success requires careful attention to risk management, trust building, human needs, team development, and workforce transformation. Join me as we explore these crucial elements of successful AI implementation and learn how to create lasting positive change in healthcare organizations.

CHAPTER 13

The Risk and Benefits of AI

The 1976 swine flu vaccination program offers crucial lessons about balancing rapid technological deployment with safety and public trust. Federal officials launched an unprecedented mass vaccination program when a new strain of influenza emerged at Fort Dix, NJ. Despite good intentions, the rushed implementation led to public concerns about vaccine safety. The federal government suspended the program after reports of Guillain-Barré syndrome emerged in vaccinated individuals. This episode parallels the challenges of implementing artificial intelligence (AI) systems in healthcare, highlighting the need for safety monitoring and transparent communication regarding its benefits and risks.

Implementing healthcare AI presents a paradox. On one side, AI technologies offer unprecedented capabilities to process vast amounts of medical data, identify patterns that might escape human observation, and automate routine tasks that consume valuable clinical time. These advantages improve patient care outcomes while reducing the administrative burden on healthcare professionals.

However, if not properly managed, these same capabilities introduce new risks to patient safety, data security, and quality of care.

Organizations must learn to harness AI's benefits while implementing robust safeguards against these risks. Comprehensive strategies that address healthcare AI's technical and operational aspects include ensuring that AI systems are appropriately trained, validated, and monitored and establishing clear protocols for use in clinical and administrative settings.

Managing Clinical Risk

Continuous testing and fostering a culture where AI augments clinical capabilities are key in managing clinical risks associated with healthcare AI. These risks manifest in various ways, from diagnostic errors to treatment recommendation failures. Successful organizations manage this risk by continuously testing the accuracy of their models and fostering a culture where AI augments clinical capabilities rather than replaces human judgment.

Organizations must establish robust policies for evaluating AI systems before implementation. These frameworks include comprehensive validation studies that assess the AI's performance across diverse patient populations and clinical scenarios. The validation process focuses on technical accuracy and evaluates the system's ability to integrate seamlessly into clinical workflows and existing IT infrastructure without introducing new sources of error.

AI systems risk generating false positives or negatives in diagnostic applications. While AI systems can enhance clinical decision-making through data analysis and pattern recognition, overreliance on these systems can lead to inappropriate treatment recommendations or missed opportunities for optimal care.

Treatment risks emerge from the complexity of clinical decision-making and the limitations of AI systems in understanding nuanced patient communication. Organizations must establish clear protocols for incorporating AI recommendations into treatment planning and implement clinical workflows supporting the primacy of clinical judgment. These recommendations include developing guidelines for when and how clinicians consider, modify, or override AI recommendations based on individual patient circumstances. Properly designed clinical workflows that lessen the probability of automation bias, where clinicians rely too heavily on AI recommendations and ignore their judgment, helps ensure that human oversight remains a central component of patient care.

Patient safety monitoring helps identify problems with AI-influenced treatment decisions. Organizations should implement strong programs for tracking treatment outcomes and identifying adverse events linked to AI-generated recommendations. These systems include establishing clear reporting mechanisms, such as incident reporting forms, regular safety meetings, and periodic reviews of treatment patterns and outcomes across different patient populations.

Healthcare professionals require comprehensive education on AI systems' capabilities and limitations. This includes understanding how to interpret AI-generated recommendations and recognize system errors while safely using AI tools.

Managing Administrative Risk

On March 28, 1979, Pennsylvania's Three Mile Island Nuclear Generating Station (TMI) experienced a partial meltdown. The incident began when a minor malfunction in the non-nuclear secondary system cascaded into automated responses, presenting the human operators with devastating information overload. The TMI operators struggled with complex interfaces, inadequate training for system-wide failures, and difficulty interpreting automated alerts. The incident led to fundamental reforms in human-machine interface design, comprehensive training protocols, and the development of a safety culture—principles directly applicable to the implementation of healthcare AI.

Healthcare AI for administrative functions presents its own set of challenges and risks. Healthcare organizations must ensure that AI systems processing patient information maintain compliance with regulatory requirements such as the Health Insurance Portability and Accountability Act (HIPAA) and the European Union's General Data Protection Regulation (GDPR). Compliance requires robust data protection measures and clear data access and handling protocols.

Administrative workflow disruption caused by introducing new AI systems can temporarily decrease efficiency as staff adapt to new processes. Organizations should carefully plan implementation timelines and provide adequate training to minimize disruptions. These measures include developing contingency plans for IT system failures or performance issues that could impact administrative functions.

Successfully integrating AI requires a careful balance between technological capability and practical usability. Healthcare organizations must ensure that AI systems enhance rather than hinder existing workflows. Workflow integration problems emerge from the disconnect between AI system capabilities and real-world needs. Redesigning workflows requires a thorough assessment that includes a detailed analysis of current processes, identification of integration points, and careful consideration of how AI tools will best support human users and interface with existing systems.

Comprehensive change management strategies help staff adapt to new AI-enhanced workflows. Organizations should provide adequate training, establish clear communication channels for feedback and support, and create mechanisms to address concerns and any resistance to change. This also includes implementing workflow efficiency and staff satisfaction monitoring systems to assess AI's impact and identify areas needing improvement.

SideBar: Obtaining a Return on Investment

Establishing clear metrics for measuring AI implementation success is crucial for ongoing optimization and justifying continued investment. Successful organizations typically track financial, operational, and clinical metrics, providing a clear roadmap for assessing the benefits of AI implementation.

Financial metrics include direct cost savings, revenue improvements, and direct and indirect benefits across multiple time periods.

Operational efficiencies typically yield short-term financial benefits. Organizations can expect administrative cost reductions within the first year of implementation, primarily through automation of routine tasks and improved resource allocation.

Medium-term returns manifest through improved clinical outcomes and reduced medical error rates. Organizations implementing AI-powered clinical decision support systems can expect reductions in length of stay and decreased readmission rates. Improved diagnostic accuracy reduces unnecessary tests and procedures.

Long-term financial benefits stem from enhanced patient outcomes, reduced liability exposure, and improved market positioning. Organizations effectively leveraging AI can increase patient satisfaction scores, improving patient retention and market share growth.

Operational metrics focus on efficiency gains, resource utilization, and process improvements. Clinical metrics track patient outcomes, error rates, and patient satisfaction.

Model Bias and Misinformation

In 1958, the tranquilizer thalidomide was first pre-scribed to pregnant women in the United Kingdom. During the three years in which it was available, approx-imately 2,000 babies were born with congenital disabili-ties. Initially tested primarily on adult male subjects, the German pharmaceutical company Chemie Grünenthal marketed the drug as a safe sedative and morning sick-ness treatment for pregnant women. The gender bias in the trials—excluding pregnant women from testing—overlooked the drug's devastating teratogenic effects, resulting in thousands of congenital disabilities world-wide. This tragedy parallels modern concerns about AI systems trained on non-representative data sets, demon-strating how sampling bias can lead to dangerous blind spots in healthcare AI systems.

The quality and representativeness of training data directly impact the performance and reliability of AI systems. Model bias, often resulting from inadequate or unrepresentative training data, leads to systematic errors that disproportionately affect specific patient populations.

Training data quality assessment should focus on technical accuracy and demographic representation. Organizations must train their AI systems on diverse datasets that reflect the characteristics of their patient population, including factors such as age, gender, ethnicity, and socioeconomic status. Regular audits of AI system performance across different patient groups help identify biases and guide corrective actions.

AI-generated content, while often accurate, can sometimes produce misleading or incorrect information that may influence clinical decision-making or a patient's understanding of their illness. Healthcare AI can generate incorrect recommendations based on incomplete or misinterpreted data. Patient-facing AI applications can provide inaccurate health information or inappropriate self-care advice. Documentation systems may generate reports with subtle but significant errors that could impact patient care decisions.

To lessen the risk of misinformation, organizations must develop comprehensive verification processes for AI-generated content that include multiple layers of human expert review. Staff training includes cross-referencing output with peer-reviewed medical knowledge and clinical guidelines.

The dynamic nature of healthcare and the evolution of AI technology necessitate continuous monitoring and improvement of AI systems. Organizations must develop processes for incorporating new medical knowledge, updated clinical guidelines, and real-world performance data into AI systems. These processes require establishing model retraining and validation protocols.

Organizations should regularly measure model performance on multiple dimensions—technical accuracy, clinical relevance, user satisfaction, and patient outcomes. This requires creating clear metrics for evaluating performance and implementing regular assessment schedules. Testing dimensions include accuracy, reliability, robustness, and fairness.

Proper maintenance of the AI model demands extensive model validation studies before implementation, regular performance assessments during operation, and specialized testing for critical updates or modifications. Organizations should also implement stress testing protocols to evaluate system performance under unusual or challenging conditions. To ensure that AI systems meet staff's practical needs, organizations must regularly assess user acceptance and provide mechanisms to obtain user feedback.

Strategic Recommendations

AI system implementation requires a structured approach to risk management. This approach begins with a comprehensive organizational readiness assessment, which includes evaluating technical infrastructure, staff capabilities, and existing processes and workflows. Organizations should establish clear objectives for AI implementation while maintaining realistic expectations about system capabilities and limitations.

Organizations need clear governance structures for overseeing AI initiatives, including designated responsibilities for risk management, performance monitoring, and system maintenance. These structures include clear lines of communication between technical teams, clinical staff, and administrative personnel.

Staff training and development are essential components of successful AI implementation. Organizations should develop comprehensive training programs that address the technical aspects of AI system operation, broader risk management, and patient safety considerations. Ongoing education programs keep staff current with system updates and emerging best practices.

Organizations should maintain detailed documentation of AI system specifications, implementation procedures, and risk management protocols, including clear guidelines for system use, error reporting, and incident response procedures. Organizational routines include regular system audits and performance reviews.

While taking these steps helps ensure successful implementations, all new technologies bring with them some risk. In my next *Bedside Consult*, I review why evaluating risk is so difficult in healthcare AI systems and the role of clinicians in mitigating that unknown risk.

Bedside Consult: Legal Liability in Healthcare— How Do We Protect Patients?

Integrating AI into healthcare heralds a new era in medical innovation. While AI offers groundbreaking potential in enhancing patient care and operational efficiency, it simultaneously introduces various legal and ethical challenges. Understanding and navigating these challenges is crucial for healthcare executives, practitioners, and AI system developers.

Complexities of Healthcare AI

AI healthcare is more than just a technological advancement; it is a transformative force reshaping patient diagnosis, treatment planning, and resource management. AI's capabilities range from predicting patient outcomes to aiding in complex surgical procedures and efficiently guiding staff and equipment use. However, the sophistication of AI systems, especially their *black-box* nature, complicates liability matters. When AI tools contribute to adverse patient outcomes, pinpointing the source of error becomes challenging. This lack of transparency in AI decision-making poses significant legal challenges, necessitating reevaluating traditional medical malpractice law and its precedents.

Managing Liability Risks

AI demands new legal frameworks that can accommodate AI's unique characteristics. Traditional medical malpractice focuses on human errors, but AI introduces errors stemming from algorithmic biases, poor choice of training data, or system failures, necessitating legal adaptability. Unlike traditional, well-documented, transparent clinical content, AI clinical content is opaque primarily due to its statistical foundation. Considering this lack of transparency, what liability do AI healthcare companies have when their software delivers poor outcomes? A promising solution to this problem is Explainable AI (XAI), which seeks to make AI decision-making processes transparent and accountable, mitigating liability risks. How XAI works continually evolves as it adapts to the increasing sophistication of AI systems.

The Indispensable Role of Clinicians

Clinicians hold a vital role in effectively utilizing AI in care delivery. Their expertise and judgment offer critical input in interpreting and contextualizing AI-generated recommendations. They ensure that AI tools complement instead of substitute for human judgment. Proper clinical workflow design incorporating AI information within the electronic health record system helps ensure that AI recommendations filter through a trained human. Furthermore, clinicians are vital in addressing privacy and ethical concerns and providing patient-centric care while navigating the techno-social landscape of healthcare AI.

Ensuring patient safety in an AI-integrated healthcare system requires a harmonious blend of technological innovation and human clinical expertise. Embedding a *human stop* within AI clinical workflows enhances patient safety by reducing the likelihood of AI-driven medical errors. In addition, clinician involvement ensures ethical AI application and patient input, maintaining the focus on patient welfare while navigating the intricacies of AI-enhanced diagnostics and treatment plans.

As AI continues to evolve and integrate deeper into healthcare, the collaboration between technology and clinical expertise becomes increasingly more critical. This collaboration is not just about enhancing healthcare delivery; it is about creating a healthcare system that is legally sound, ethically responsible, and focused on patient welfare. Future developments in healthcare AI healthcare must consider these issues, ensuring that the legal frameworks, ethical guidelines, and clinical practices evolve with technological change.

Healthcare artificial intelligence necessitates forward-thinking approaches to risk management and system optimization. As technology develops and becomes more deeply integrated into healthcare delivery systems, new forms of risk may arise. This requires the development of adaptive risk management strategies to accommodate these evolving challenges. Healthcare organizations that successfully manage the risks of healthcare AI are better positioned to leverage these technologies for improved patient care and operational efficiency.

CHAPTER 14

Aligning AI with Human Needs

In 1847, Hungarian physician Dr. Ignaz Semmelweis made a groundbreaking discovery that would eventually transform medical practice: handwashing significantly reduced maternal mortality rates. While working at the Vienna General Hospital, Semmelweis observed that physicians who disinfected their hands with a chlorinated lime solution before delivering babies drastically reduced the incidence of puerperal fever, a leading cause of maternal deaths due to infection. Despite presenting clear, evidence-backed results, his findings were met with resistance from the medical establishment, which was reluctant to accept the notion that unwashed hands transmitted disease. It took decades—and the advent of germ theory through Louis Pasteur and Joseph Lister— for Semmelweis's life-saving practice to gain widespread acceptance, cementing its role in modern hygiene and infection control.

Technological advancements bring new challenges. The increasing sophistication of artificial intelligence (AI) models raises questions about interpretability, biases, and the need for robust validation due to their use in clinical settings. As AI systems become more autonomous in their decision-making capabilities, healthcare organizations must address questions of accountability and strike an appropriate balance between AI assistance and human judgment.

Healthcare organizations should ensure that their AI systems' behaviors and outputs align with human intentions and ethical standards. This alignment problem is a theoretical concern that is a real issue that directly impacts patient well-being, safety, and societal costs. The ethical deployment of AI technologies necessitates strict adherence to Hippocrates' principle of *do no harm*.

Organizations can address this alignment problem by embedding ethical, transparent, and rights-focused principles into their AI strategies. The U.S. government's call for an *AI Bill of Rights* underscores the need for a comprehensive approach to address healthcare AI use. This framework prioritizes patient safety, safeguarding privacy, and actively combating bias within AI algorithms.

Transparency in AI operations and decision-making processes is essential for building and maintaining patient trust. Patients deserve a clear understanding of how their data influences AI-driven clinical decisions and drives patient care. The American Medical Association advocates for clear communication in AI system deployment, ensuring patients and practitioners comprehend how AI tools function and obtain information on bias in its recommendations.

AI Safety Institutes

Developing and implementing safe AI technologies necessitate collaborative approaches through public-private partnerships to increase the probability of success. Establishing AI safety institutes brings together government agencies, private sector companies, academic institutions, and non-profits to focus on research and development to ensure the safe deployment of AI technologies.

These partnerships are crucial in addressing complex challenges such as bias detection, privacy preservation, and the creation of standardized frameworks for assessing and mitigating risk. Through pooled resources and expertise, organizations can tackle challenges too vast for any single entity to handle.

Regular engagement with patients and community stakeholders ensures AI implementations meet public expectations and needs. This engagement includes clear communication about how AI systems influence care decisions and what safeguards exist to protect patient interests. Organizations should establish clear channels for stakeholder feedback and demonstrate responsiveness to concerns raised about AI systems.

Like the **CE** marking indicating a product has met all European Union specifications, healthcare organizations and technology vendors should implement comprehensive validation processes to verify that their AI systems meet predetermined safety and efficacy standards. These standards include testing in various clinical settings with representative patient populations to identify and mitigate biases or limitations before widespread deployment.

Similar to technical notes issued during new software releases, vendors should publish detailed reports on every major update of their healthcare AI tools. Reports with focused updates for specialty clinicians and patients will build needed trust.

As healthcare organizations work to align AI systems with human needs, implementing robust monitoring systems becomes increasingly important. Just as the pharmaceutical industry developed pharmacovigilance to monitor drug safety after the thalidomide tragedy of the 1950s, healthcare must now establish similar vigilance systems for AI algorithms. The concept of algorithmovigilance represents this essential evolution in healthcare safety monitoring.

Side Bar: Algorithmovigilance and Safety Monitoring

Only robust monitoring systems can adequately evaluate the effectiveness of AI systems' ongoing safety and impact on care. *Algorithmovigilance*, focusing on continuous monitoring and analysis of AI systems, is a critical tool for detecting and correcting any *drifts* in models that may occur over time due to evolving patient demographics and changes in the data used for model training.

Healthcare professionals are responsible for interpreting AI-generated results that influence patient care. This stewardship requires considering biases and disparities in the data used to train AI models. By equipping healthcare providers with the knowledge and skills to oversee AI systems and understand their capabilities and limitations, organizations ensure that the use of AI systems aligns with ethical standards and patient needs.

Implementing *AI safety nets* is a major component of algorithmic stewardship. These protocols and systems catch errors or inappropriate recommendations before they impact patient care. Organizations may employ secondary AI systems to cross-check primary AI outputs or implement structured human review processes for high-stakes decisions.

Establishing Development Standards

In 1928, Sir Alexander Fleming's accidental discovery of penicillin led to a revolution in medicine. Still, it was only in the structured development and testing standards established by Dr. Howard Florey and Ernst Chain in 1941 that this powerful tool could be safely deployed at scale. Their systematic approach to drug development and safety testing created the foundation for modern pharmaceutical standards. Similarly, healthcare organizations today must develop rigorous AI develop-

ment and deployment standards to ensure these powerful tools serve their intended purpose safely and effectively.

These comprehensive standards, or constitutions, codify core
values and norms governing AI development and implementation.
These constitutions guide developers and help ensure AI systems
adhere to ethical standards and regulatory requirements while safeguarding patient well-being and privacy.

The guidance should address several critical areas, including
transparency in operations, accountability for outcomes, and equity
in healthcare delivery. Periodic assessment of AI systems against
these constitutional principles ensures ongoing alignment with strategic objectives and organizational responsibilities. Organizations
must also test their AI systems across various scenarios, particularly
those mimicking real-world clinical environments, and customize
them to the uniqueness of their patient population.

Establishing clear protocols for human oversight ensures
AI systems augment rather than replace clinical judgment. This
approach includes realistic clinical workflows that facilitate clinician review of AI-generated recommendations and implementing
fail-safe mechanisms to modulate AI system functions if dangerous
outcomes are detected.

Successful organizations move beyond simple explainability
to achieve true *interpretability* in their AI systems. While explainability focuses on making AI outputs understandable, interpretability enables clinicians to comprehend the underlying factors and
decision-making processes. This deeper understanding is crucial in
complex clinical scenarios where simple explanations or visual aids
do not suffice.

Implementing layered explanations allows users to explore AI decisions at multiple levels of complexity. Organizations should develop interactive tools that enable clinicians to query specific aspects of AI recommendations and understand how different factors influence outcomes. This approach helps build trust in AI systems, enabling more informed clinical decision-making. A similar approach is also valuable in deploying chatbots and other AI tools that interface with patients.

Healthcare AI deployment without appropriate regulations leads to unintended consequences that undermine patient trust and safety. Although for-profit motives facilitate innovation, they sometimes conflict with society's interests. The extent of regulation can impact innovation, requiring regulatory bodies to develop carefully crafted rules that protect patients while not slowing technological advancement.

Identifying areas that can most benefit from innovation while maintaining strong ethical standards requires collaboration by a broad group of stakeholders, including clinicians, ethicists, data scientists, patient advocates, and technology leaders. Clinicians serve as custodians of patient care and trust, making their insights invaluable in shaping AI tools.

Healthcare organizations and technology vendors must navigate complex intellectual property issues as they develop and implement AI solutions. Large language models present unique challenges in intellectual property law, particularly regarding using training data and protecting proprietary information. In addition, organizations must determine how to fairly share financial gains with the many stakeholders who contribute to the AI tool's development. AI companies in every market face claims from content creators who seek compensation for using their content to train AI models. In healthcare, the patient is the most valuable content creator, and how to compensate them is complex and controversial.

The balance between encouraging market entry and protecting developer and content creator rights requires careful consideration. Clear guidance is needed to allow innovation and protect intellectual property rights while ensuring continued innovation and a competitive marketplace.

Organizations must prepare for the continued evolution of AI capabilities and applications. Advances in federated learning, quantum computing, and neuromorphic systems that mimic the functioning of the human brain will create new opportunities and challenges for AI in healthcare delivery.

AI systems' theoretical frameworks and technical implementations ultimately converge on a fundamental question—How do we protect individual rights and privacy in an era of unprecedented data utilization? My next *Bedside Consult* explores this critical intersection of progress and privacy, examining the parallels between tech industry practices and healthcare data usage.

Bedside Consult: The Price of Progress—Protecting Patient Privacy in the Age of AI

As AI continues to revolutionize industries across the globe, its impact on healthcare is becoming increasingly apparent. From diagnosis and treatment planning to drug discovery and clinical trials, AI has the potential to transform patient care and clinical outcomes. However, this rapid advancement has also raised significant concerns about using protected health information (PHI) stored in electronic health records without obtaining prior patient permission.

In *The New York Times* article "How Tech Giants Cut Corners to Harvest Data for AI," Metz et al. (2024) shed light on a similar issue in the tech industry. Companies like OpenAI, Google, and Meta have been using copyrighted material without permission to train their AI models, sparking debates about intellectual property rights and to the ethical use of data in the AI age. OpenAI, in particular, faced a data shortage in late 2021 and resorted to transcribing over one million hours of YouTube videos, violating the platform's terms of service. Similarly, Google used YouTube video transcripts to train its AI models despite the unclear legal and ethical implications.

Running Out of Data

Tech companies are growing concerned about the scarcity of new high-quality data for training AI models. As the demand for data increases, companies are looking for new sources, including copyrighted material and user-generated content, and even considering the acquisition of publishing houses like Simon & Schuster to gain access to long-form text. The debate around fair use and the need for licensing data has become contentious, with some arguing that the scale required for AI development makes traditional licensing impractical.

Furthermore, access to data in the AI race remains a critical component as researchers emphasize that *scale is all you need* when training large language models. The competition for data to create more powerful AI tools has led to a rapid increase in the size of training datasets, from hundreds of billions of tokens to trillions of tokens in just a few years. As a result, tech companies are exploring alternative data sources, including generating synthetic data using AI models. In AI, a token is a fundamental unit of data in an extensive data set, such as a word, character, or phrase, processed by algorithms.

Synthetic Data

Synthetic data is generated by AI models rather than collected from real-world sources. Tech companies like OpenAI believe that synthetic data could be the solution to the looming data shortage. By training AI models to generate realistic text, images, and other forms of data, companies hope to create a self-sustaining loop where AI can learn from its outputs. However, this approach is challenging, as AI-generated data may lack the diversity and quality necessary for robust model training. Misinformation in data sets used to train synthetic AI models could create a feedback loop that generates more and more misinformation and poor-quality AI. Despite these concerns, synthetic data will likely become more prevalent as tech companies seek to maintain their competitive edge.

Copyright and PHI Parallels

The parallels between using copyrighted material in the tech industry and using PHI in healthcare are striking. Patients, by law, own and have control over their medical records. This fundamental right was codified by law to protect individual privacy and maintain trust between patients and healthcare providers. Traditionally, when medical researchers seek to use patient data for studies, they obtain written permission from every participant. This process ensures transparency and allows patients to decide how researchers can use their personal information.

However, the widespread adoption of electronic health record systems has created a vast repository of digital health data, which is irresistible to researchers and companies developing AI tools. Like the issue faced by the tech industry using copyrighted material to train their AI models, using electronic health record data has sparked debates about intellectual property rights and the ethical use of PHI without permission.

Consent Required

In healthcare, the stakes are even higher. PHI is not copyrighted; it is sensitive information directly impacting patients' lives and well-being. When organizations use this data without consent, it erodes the trust between patients and the healthcare system. Moreover, it raises questions about the ownership and control of personal health data in our increasingly digital world.

Some argue that de-identifying patient data is sufficient to protect privacy and justify its use in AI development. However, this argument fails to address the fundamental issue of patient consent. Even if developers strip personally identifiable information from the data, it belongs to the patient who generated it. Using this data without permission violates patient autonomy and breaches trust.

Regulations Controlling Use

Developing healthcare AI tools requires vast amounts of diverse, high-quality data to ensure accuracy and reliability. While obtaining individual consent from every patient may be impractical, the need for guidelines and regulations governing the use of PHI in AI research and product development is still relevant.

These guidelines must prioritize patient privacy and ensure that the use of data directly benefits patient care. One approach is establishing a framework where for-profit organizations accessing patient data contribute a portion of their profits to non-profit entities dedicated to advancing the public good. These funds can support AI research grants, clinical trials, or other initiatives that directly improve patient outcomes. A public-private partnership offers another path forward.

Additionally, patients should be able to opt in or out of having their data used for AI development. This can be achieved through clear, concise consent forms that explain how the data will be used, who will have access to it, and what benefits, if any, will be shared with patients. Transparency and patient engagement are vital to building trust and fostering a collaborative approach to AI in healthcare.

It is crucial to balance enabling AI innovation and protecting patient rights. The goal is not to stifle progress but to ensure it happens ethically and responsibly. By involving patients in the process and ensuring that they benefit from the use of their data, we can create a healthcare system that leverages the power of AI while maintaining the highest standards of privacy and trust.

Informed Consent

As we navigate this new frontier of AI in healthcare, we must have open and honest conversations about data ownership, consent, and responsible use of PHI. Patients, healthcare providers, researchers, policymakers, and industry leaders must collaborate to develop a framework that promotes innovation while safeguarding patient rights.

The potential benefits of AI in healthcare are immense—from early detection of diseases to personalized treatment plans and improved outcomes. However, we must not lose sight of the human element at the core of this endeavor. Patients are not just data points; they have the right to control their health information.

By prioritizing patient consent, fostering transparency, and ensuring that AI's benefits are shared equitably, we can harness the power of this technology to transform healthcare for the better. Our collective responsibility is to build a future where AI and patient rights coexist harmoniously, paving the way for a healthier, more empowered society.

The lessons learned from the tech industry's struggle with data usage and intellectual property rights serve as a cautionary tale for the healthcare sector. As we embrace the potential of AI in medicine, we must proactively address the ethical and legal challenges surrounding patient data. By engaging in open dialogue, establishing clear guidelines, and prioritizing patient rights, we can ensure that the integration of AI in healthcare is both innovative and responsible, ultimately benefiting patients and society.

Healthcare organizations must strike a delicate balance: embracing the transformative power of artificial intelligence while maintaining rigorous standards for safety, transparency, and ethical deployment. By establishing comprehensive frameworks for development, implementing robust monitoring systems, and maintaining clear communication with all stakeholders, organizations can create AI systems that genuinely serve human needs. The future of healthcare AI depends not only on technical advancement but on our ability to align these powerful tools with the fundamental values of medicine: beneficence, non-maleficence, justice, and respect for human autonomy.

CHAPTER 15

Trust, Distrust, and Hallucinations

On October 30, 1938, Orson Welles' radio adaptation of "War of the Worlds" presented a fictional alien invasion through simulated news bulletins. The broadcast created widespread panic among listeners who accepted it as truth despite clear disclaimers about its fictional nature. The aftermath brought intense media scrutiny, with newspapers and public figures condemning the broadcast's news-bulletin format as deliberately deceptive.

Effective use of artificial intelligence (AI) depends upon establishing and maintaining trust between humans and AI tools. Organizations cultivate and sustain trust among healthcare professionals, patients, and regulatory bodies by following transparent, ethical, and responsible practices.

Errors or misinformation in healthcare AI—often termed *hallucinations*—directly affect patient safety and outcomes. A misdiagnosis suggested by an AI system, an incorrect medication recommendation, or a flawed treatment plan can lead to serious harm.

The primary requirement for using healthcare AI lies in understanding that trust is not inherent in these systems—it must be actively built and maintained. Healthcare organizations must ensure that professionals and patients understand AI's capabilities and limitations. This understanding requires clear communication about how AI algorithms work, what data they use, and how their outputs are interpreted and applied.

Building trust demands more than technical training for clinicians. It requires creating an environment where clinicians feel confident using AI content alongside their clinical judgment. Clinicians should learn when to rely on AI recommendations and when to reject them based on clinical expertise.

Patients deserve the confidence that organizations use their health information appropriately and that AI-driven recommendations serve their best interests. This requires transparency in AI's role in their care, clear explanations of how their data is protected, and assurance that human oversight remains central to all clinical decisions.

Understanding AI Hallucinations

AI is nothing more than a mathematical model stuffed with probabilities calculated by ingesting vast amounts of data. Adjusting the model's parameters and curating training data determines an AI system's usefulness and power. Unlike human intelligence, AI possesses no knowledge, ethics, or opinions. Healthcare AI hallucinations are outputs or recommendations generated by statistical probabilities, like all AI content, but are not grounded in the real world or supported by underlying data. These hallucinations can manifest in various ways:

- A diagnostic AI system might identify patterns that do not exist, leading to false positive results.
- A clinical documentation system might generate detailed but fictional patient histories.

- A treatment recommendation system might suggest therapies based on misinterpreted or non-existent clinical evidence.

The consequences of such hallucinations erode trust in AI systems, harming patients if not identified and corrected, and create liability issues for healthcare and vendor organizations. Understanding why hallucinations occur is crucial for managing these risks.

AI hallucinations often stem from limitations in training data, gaps in the model's knowledge base, or the inherent uncertainties in machine learning (ML) algorithms. When an AI system encounters situations that differ significantly from its training data, it may attempt to generate responses based on incomplete or incorrect pattern matching, leading to plausible but dangerous outputs. AI always tries to *please you* by responding, even if that response is fabricated gibberish.

Robust evaluation and testing protocols prevent AI hallucinations and maintain system reliability. Just as clinical trials validate new treatments before implementation, AI systems require rigorous and frequent assessment to ensure safety and effectiveness.

Sidebar: Evaluation and Testing

Successful organizations regularly assess the completeness and accuracy of model training data while remaining vigilant for biases affecting AI performance. This ongoing attention to data quality helps prevent many common sources of AI hallucinations and response errors.

The dynamic nature of AI systems demands ongoing evaluation and monitoring, an essential defense against AI errors. Monitoring programs that track performance metrics, safety indicators, user feedback, and system updates using technical data combined with human oversight lessens the chance of hallucinations. This monitoring should also assess AI system accuracy, reliability, and consistency across patient populations and clinical scenarios.

The intensity of system verification should match the level of risk associated with the AI application. High-stakes decisions, such as invasive or costly diagnostic or treatment recommendations, require multiple levels of verification, including review by specialists and multidisciplinary teams.

Healthcare providers represent a crucial source of insight into AI system performance. Their daily interaction with these systems places them in an ideal position to identify problems. By creating effective channels for collecting and analyzing feedback, organizations can use it to improve system performance and prevent future errors.

Organizations must respond swiftly and systematically when identifying AI errors or hallucinations. This response begins with immediate actions to protect patient safety, including correcting affected records and notifying relevant clinicians and patients. However, effective response protocols extend beyond immediate corrections to include a thorough investigation of root causes, implementation of preventive measures, and notification of vendors and other stakeholders.

Each significant error or hallucination presents an opportunity for system improvement. By carefully analyzing these incidents, organizations can identify patterns, refine their AI systems, and strengthen their verification processes. This systematic approach to learning from errors helps prevent similar issues from recurring while continuously improving system reliability.

Regulations and Oversight

In 1982, seven people died after consuming cyanide-laced capsules of Extra Strength Tylenol purchased in the Chicago area. Soon after other incidents around the country, Johnson & Johnson, the maker of Tylenol, recalled all 31 million bottles in circulation, representing over $100 million of inventory. Johnson & Johnson's transparent response—including the first nationwide product recall and development of tamper-proof packaging—set new standards for corporate responsibility and safety protocols.

Regulation of healthcare AI continues to evolve as technology advances and understanding of risks deepens. While innovation often outpaces regulation, several key regulatory bodies oversee and govern healthcare AI implementation.

The U.S. regulatory approach for healthcare AI involves multiple federal agencies overseeing different aspects of AI implementation and use. The U.S. Food and Drug Administration (FDA) is the most prominent agency, pivotal in regulating AI-based medical devices and software.

Under current FDA frameworks, AI systems directly influencing patient care decisions are typically classified as medical devices. The level of regulatory oversight depends on the intended use and risk to patients. High-risk AI applications, such as diagnostic recommendations or therapeutic guidance, face more stringent requirements than lower-risk applications used for administrative purposes.

The FDA proposed a new regulatory framework for AI/ML-based Software as a Medical Device, acknowledging that these technologies require ongoing monitoring and assessment throughout their lifecycle. This framework emphasizes the importance of real-world performance monitoring and the need for predetermined change control plans that allow algorithm updates while maintaining safety and effectiveness.

The *regulatory sandbox* concept, controlled environments where organizations can test innovative AI technologies under regulatory supervision, provides space for experimentation while ensuring compliance with safety and ethical standards.

The Centers for Medicare & Medicaid Services (CMS) influences the adoption of healthcare AI through its coverage and reimbursement decisions. The agency's expanding role in health technology assessment directly impacts how healthcare organizations implement and utilize AI systems. CMS has begun developing frameworks for evaluating AI technologies' clinical effectiveness and value, which will increasingly influence which AI tools gain widespread adoption.

The U.S. Federal Trade Commission (FTC) is another important regulatory body focused on consumer protection. The agency works to prevent deceptive practices and ensure that AI applications do not mislead consumers or violate privacy rights. This oversight extends to marketing claims about AI capabilities and the accuracy of AI-generated health information.

The FTC's role becomes particularly relevant in addressing AI hallucinations and misinformation, as the agency has the authority to take action against organizations that fail to prevent or address harmful AI-generated content that could impact public health or consumer safety.

Recent executive orders, particularly "Executive Order 14110" (Executive Office of the President, 2023), significantly shape the regulatory landscape. These orders emphasize the need for robust AI assurance policies and infrastructure to measure AI models' pre-market and postmarket performance against real-world data. They also call for developing standards and guidelines to harness AI capabilities while minimizing associated risks.

The executive orders catalyzed efforts to create more comprehensive regulatory frameworks, pushing agencies to develop new approaches for evaluating and monitoring AI systems throughout their lifecycle. These approaches include requirements for ongoing performance monitoring, bias detection, and regular reassessment of AI systems' safety and effectiveness.

Beyond federal oversight, individual states began implementing AI regulations, creating a complex patchwork of requirements that healthcare organizations must navigate. States like Illinois and California are leading in establishing AI governance frameworks regarding privacy protection and transparency requirements.

While necessary for protecting consumers and patients, this state-level activity challenges healthcare organizations operating across multiple jurisdictions. This factor requires organizations to design their AI governance to comply with the most stringent applicable regulations while maintaining flexibility to adapt to evolving requirements across different jurisdictions.

European Union's Approach to AI

The European Union (EU) takes a distinctly different approach to AI regulation, implementing a comprehensive, risk-based framework that directly and indirectly affects healthcare AI applications. This approach fundamentally differs from the U.S. model by establishing horizontal rules that apply across sectors while maintaining specific requirements for healthcare applications.

At the center of European AI regulation stands the Artificial Intelligence Act (AIA), which establishes a hierarchical, risk-based approach to AI oversight. This framework categorizes AI systems based on their risk level, with healthcare applications frequently falling into the high-risk category due to their impact on human health and safety.

Under the AIA, healthcare AI systems face rigorous requirements for:

- Data quality and governance
- Technical documentation and record-keeping

- Transparency and user information
- Human oversight
- Accuracy, robustness, and cybersecurity
- Risk management systems

The European Medicines Agency complements the AIA framework by providing specific guidance for AI applications in medical devices and pharmaceutical development. The agency emphasizes continuous monitoring and validation of AI systems, particularly those influencing clinical decision-making or directing patient care.

Preparing for Rapid Change

In 1911, Frederick Winslow Taylor's publication of "The Principles of Scientific Management" marked a pivotal shift in how organizations approached process verification. Taylor established the revolutionary concept that every industrial process could be broken down, measured, and systematically verified. His methods faced fierce resistance from workers who saw this data-driven approach as dehumanizing. Despite this resistance, Taylor's principles laid the foundation for modern quality control systems and demonstrated how systematic measurement could improve reliability.

Organizations implementing AI systems must develop comprehensive compliance strategies that address multiple regulatory frameworks. These strategies require the development of flexible governance structures that adapt to evolving requirements while maintaining consistent standards across all operations. Organizations should remain proactive in developing and refining their compliance strategies rather than waiting for regulatory requirements to drive change.

International organizations may need to develop systems that can simultaneously satisfy the documentation requirements of the FDA, meet the risk management standards of the EU's AIA, and address state-specific regulations in the United States. This complexity often necessitates creating centralized AI governance teams that coordinate compliance efforts across jurisdictions.

Vital technical considerations include:

Real-World Performance Monitoring: The establishment of robust systems for tracking AI performance across different populations and contexts, ensuring that systems maintain their safety and effectiveness over time.

Documentation and Traceability: Creating regulatory frameworks that emphasize the importance of comprehensive documentation of AI system development, testing, and ongoing performance and require organizations to implement systems that track decisions and changes throughout the AI system lifecycle.

Bias Detection and Mitigation: Regularly assess AI systems for biases and implement corrective measures when necessary, documenting these efforts to satisfy regulatory requirements.

The regulatory landscape continues to evolve rapidly as technology advances and understanding of risks improves. The growth of personalized medicine and precision healthcare requires AI tools to communicate with each other to generate increasingly specific recommendations based on individual patient characteristics. As organizations move to deploy multiple AI tools that communicate with each other, the probability of cascading errors or compound hallucinations increases. These trends amplify the importance of maintaining robust verification processes while ensuring AI systems appropriately handle unique or unusual cases without generating hallucinations or errors.

Organizations must remain adaptable and anticipate more stringent regulations as AI capabilities expand. Several trends appear likely to shape future regulatory developments:

Increased Focus on Explainability: Regulators will emphasize the ability to explain AI decision-making processes, particularly in high-stakes healthcare applications.

Enhanced Postmarket Surveillance: Requirements for monitoring AI performance after deployment will become more rigorous, emphasizing real-world evidence and outcomes.

International Harmonization: Efforts to align regulatory frameworks across jurisdictions will increase, reducing the complexity of compliance for global organizations.

Technology vendors, healthcare providers, regulatory bodies, and patients must collaborate more closely to develop integrated AI safety and reliability strategies. This collaboration should extend to sharing data about AI performance, errors, and successful risk management approaches while maintaining appropriate privacy and security protections.

The theoretical frameworks and regulatory considerations for managing AI trust and preventing hallucinations ensure that healthcare AI always serves the best interests of patients and society. In my next *Bedside Consult*, I suggest ways to achieve that objective.

Bedside Consult: Beyond Black Box Healthcare AI—Gain Trust with Transparency

The rapid advancement of AI in healthcare has ushered in a new era of possibilities, promising improved patient outcomes, enhanced operational efficiency, and groundbreaking research. This wave of innovation brings with it a sense of optimism and excitement for the future of healthcare. However, as we stand at this technological crossroads, it is crucial to establish robust frameworks for developing, testing, and maintaining AI systems.

November 2022 marked a significant milestone in the public's experience with AI, as ChatGPT demonstrated the capabilities of large language models to millions of users worldwide. This event catalyzed discussions about the applications of generative AI in various sectors, including healthcare. Unlike traditional predictive AI models, generative AI, or GenAI, produces natural language outputs, making it a form of relational AI that can interact with users in more human-like ways.

The applications of GenAI in healthcare are vast and promising. From drafting patient-portal messages to creating conversational interfaces for patient education and even facilitating preliminary self-diagnosis, GenAI could revolutionize how healthcare information is communicated and accessed. However, this new frontier of AI also brings a host of ethical considerations that must be carefully addressed.

Ethical Considerations

In their *New England Journal of Medicine* article, "The ethics of relational AI—Expanding and implementing the Belmont Principles," Sim and Cassel (2024) note that the introduction of AI-generated text, speech, images, and video between clinicians and patients fundamentally alters the ethical landscape of healthcare delivery. Physicians' traditional fiduciary responsibility to uphold principles of beneficence, respect for persons, and justice now extends to the AI systems they use.

The ethical implementation of AI in healthcare demands that these systems be Fair, Appropriate, Valid, Effective, and Safe. However, ensuring adherence to these principles is challenging due to AI's complex nature. Large language models' probabilistic nature introduces inherent errors or hallucination risks, which could have severe consequences in a healthcare setting.

Moreover, the potential for AI systems to pursue goal-oriented behavior misaligned with medical ethics—such as optimizing for insurer profits rather than patient outcomes—underscores the need for rigorous ethical oversight. As healthcare leaders, we must ensure that AI systems prioritize patient benefit above all else, followed by considerations for providers and broader society.

The Call for AI Assurance Laboratories

There is a growing consensus on the need for a nationwide network of healthcare AI assurance laboratories to address the potential problems of AI. In their *JAMA* article, "A nationwide network of health AI assurance laboratories," Shah et al. (2024) proposed that these labs would be shared resources for validating AI models, accelerating responsible innovation, and ensuring safe deployment in healthcare settings.

These assurance labs would provide comprehensive evaluations of AI models, ranging from technical performance assessments to analyses of biases and simulations of real-world effects. By offering different levels of evaluation, from basic technical validations to in-depth assessments of usability and adoption via human-machine teaming, these labs could provide crucial insights into the benefits and risks of AI systems before their deployment in clinical settings.

Creating such a network would promote transparency and accountability in AI development. By publishing evaluation results openly in a nationwide registry, these labs would enable healthcare providers, policymakers, and the public to make informed decisions about the use of AI in healthcare. In addition, the labs form a repository of knowledge on developing, testing, and deploying AI in various healthcare settings with different overall goals.

The Need for Ongoing Monitoring and Revalidation

Robust AI assurance requires continuous monitoring and revalidation of AI models. Unlike traditional medical interventions, AI systems can *drift* over time, leading to degraded performance or unexpected behaviors and, in turn, undesirable outcomes. This issue is particularly relevant for generative AI models, which may be updated or fine-tuned regularly.

As a result, we must establish processes for managing AI models' lifecycles to ensure they maintain their performance over time across diverse populations and in various clinical settings. This ongoing monitoring, which includes regular revalidation, is a precaution and a reassurance that we are committed to identifying and mitigating harms before they impact patient care.

Transparency and Ethical Imperatives

While GenAI offers tremendous benefits to patients and providers, we must establish stringent standards for its development, testing, and maintenance. These standards include a strong emphasis on transparency. Black box AI systems, where there is no transparency into the algorithms used, training data, or steps taken to prevent harm, are unacceptable in healthcare. By ensuring transparency, we keep all stakeholders informed and involved in the evolution of healthcare AI.

We should prioritize the development of interpretable and explainable AI models that allow for meaningful oversight and accountability. This transparency is crucial for regulatory compliance and building trust among patients, providers, and the public.

Furthermore, we must be wary of perverse incentives that may arise when testing is left solely to AI developers. As Sim and Cassel point out, there is a risk of AI systems optimized for outcomes that benefit insurers or other stakeholders at the expense of patient care or provider autonomy. Independent assurance laboratories and ongoing third-party evaluations are essential to mitigate this risk.

As we integrate AI into healthcare, we must do so with a steadfast commitment to ethical principles and patient safety. Establishing a nationwide network of health AI assurance laboratories, coupled with robust standards for ongoing monitoring and revalidation, is crucial in realizing AI's potential while mitigating its risks.

Leadership requires healthcare professionals to actively participate in shaping the future of AI in medicine, advocating for transparency, ethical development, and rigorous evaluation. By doing so, we can ensure that AI is a powerful tool to enhance patient care, support healthcare providers, and ultimately improve health outcomes for all.

The evolution of healthcare artificial intelligence mirrors many historical transitions in medicine—from the initial excitement of innovation to the sobering recognition of risks and the eventual development of balanced, evidence-based approaches to implementation. As we expand our use of AI in delivering patient care, we must learn from history's lessons about the importance of systematic validation, transparent operations, and robust safety measures. Successful implementation of AI technologies depends on technological capabilities and our ability to build and maintain trust through careful oversight, continuous monitoring, and unwavering commitment to patient safety. The future of healthcare AI lies not in blind adoption or excessive caution but in thoughtful integration that balances innovation with responsibility.

CHAPTER 16

Building Teams and Effecting Change

In April 1970, the Apollo XIII mission faced a catastrophic oxygen tank explosion, leaving the spacecraft crippled 200,000 miles from Earth. NASA Flight Director Gene Kranz led a multidisciplinary team of engineers, scientists, and astronauts in a high-pressure effort to devise innovative solutions using only the spacecraft's limited resources. Among their critical achievements was the creation of a makeshift carbon dioxide scrubber from spare parts, ensuring the crew's survival. Kranz's leadership, characterized by clear communication, rapid problem-solving, and an unwavering commitment to success, embodied in the phrase *failure is not an option*, played a pivotal role in safely returning the crew to Earth. Fueled by their determination, this extraordinary collaboration set a standard for solving complex challenges under pressure, offering valuable lessons for modern technical teams.

Most healthcare organizations recognize that successfully implementing healthcare artificial intelligence (AI) is not just about acquiring and deploying sophisticated technology. It is about orchestrating diverse expertise, developing new skill sets, and, most importantly, forming cohesive interdisciplinary teams. These teams bridge the gap between clinical knowledge and technological capabilities, making unique expertise and perspectives crucial to the success of healthcare AI.

The concept of prompt engineering emerges as a crucial link in this collaborative chain. Prompt engineering, the sophisticated art and science of crafting inputs that guide AI systems to produce desired outcomes, is the primary mechanism by which healthcare professionals advance the capabilities of healthcare AI. However, developing effective prompts requires more than technical expertise; it demands a deep understanding of clinical workflows, medical terminology, and the nuanced decision-making processes that characterize healthcare delivery. Combining subject matter expertise with the knowledge of creating high-quality prompts is the most effective way to safely and effectively create practical healthcare AI systems.

The Art and Science of Prompt Engineering

The design of effective AI-driven clinical decision support systems requires close collaboration between clinical experts and technical teams. These systems must not only provide accurate information but must do so in ways that enhance rather than disrupt workflows.

Developing effective prompts requires careful attention to how healthcare professionals approach clinical problems. Prompt engineers must work closely with clinicians to understand what information is needed and how to present that information to be most beneficial for the clinician at the point of care.

Successful organizations approach this challenge through detailed mapping of clinical decision-making processes. This mapping identifies critical decision points where AI support can provide the most value while ensuring system responses align with clinical thinking patterns.

Prompt engineering goes beyond simple query construction. It requires careful consideration of clinical context, patient safety implications, and the complex decision-making processes inherent in care delivery. For instance, when developing prompts for diagnostic support systems, engineers must consider the presenting symptoms and the broader context of patient history, risk factors, and potential complications. The latest clinical evidence, as documented in journal articles and curated by organization experts, enhances the model's responses.

The process begins with close collaboration between clinical experts and prompt engineers to define the AI system's precise requirements to generate the desired outcomes. Clinical experts provide crucial insights into decision-making processes while prompt engineers translate these insights into structured inputs that effectively guide AI systems. This collaborative approach ensures prompts elicit technically accurate, clinically relevant, and safe actionable responses.

Sidebar: Building Interdisciplinary Excellence

Interdisciplinary collaboration is a beneficial aspect and the cornerstone of successful healthcare AI. It brings together diverse expertise and perspectives, creating teams that can effectively direct healthcare AI systems' creation, deployment, and evolution. These teams typically include:

Clinical Specialists: Bring deep domain knowledge and understanding of patient care requirements. Their expertise ensures that AI implementations align with clinical needs and workflows while maintaining the highest standards of patient care.

Prompt Engineers: Possess the technical expertise to craft and refine the instructions that guide AI systems. These specialists bridge clinical requirements and technological capabilities, translating medical knowledge into effective AI interactions.

Data Scientists: Contribute their understanding of AI algorithms, data structures, and analytics. Their expertise ensures that AI systems process and analyze healthcare data accurately and effectively.

AI Ethicists: Provide crucial oversight regarding the ethical implications of AI implementation. Their role includes identifying biases, ensuring patient privacy, and maintaining ethical standards of patient care.

Healthcare Informaticists: Understand both clinical processes and information technology systems. Their expertise proves invaluable in integrating AI solutions with existing healthcare information systems and workflows.

The success of these interdisciplinary teams depends on developing shared understanding and effective communication channels. Each team member must understand other disciplines' perspectives and requirements, creating a foundation for effective collaboration.

Frameworks for Effective Collaboration

In 1942, J. Robert Oppenheimer faced the immense challenge of leading the Los Alamos Laboratory as part of the Manhattan Project, coordinating a diverse team of over 6,000 personnel, including Nobel laureates, scientists, engineers, and military staff. His innovative leadership included establishing a coordinating council for division leaders, fostering interdisciplinary communication, and creating informal forums like colloquium series to encourage collaboration across disciplines. By balancing scientific autonomy with project objectives, Oppenheimer successfully managed one of history's most complex technical endeavors, demonstrating how structured knowledge-sharing and team interaction are essential for large-scale innovation.

Successful knowledge-sharing programs include regular workshops where clinicians explain complex medical decision-making processes to technical team members. In turn, technical experts demonstrate the capabilities and limitations of AI systems to clinical staff.

Clear communication and a common vocabulary facilitate effective collaboration. Teams develop strategies to bridge the linguistic and conceptual gaps between clinical and technical domains, creating a shared understanding that fosters effective problem-solving.

Beyond structured environments, successful organizations implement mentoring systems where experienced team members from different disciplines work closely together, sharing insights and developing a deeper appreciation for each other's domains. This approach helps break down traditional silos, fostering more innovative and effective solutions.

※

Leading AI-driven healthcare organizations create structured frameworks for collaboration that address the unique challenges of healthcare AI development and deployment. These frameworks typically incorporate several key elements:

Structured Communication: Protocols establish clear channels and methodologies for sharing information between clinical and technical team members. These protocols ensure critical information flows effectively across disciplinary boundaries, highlighting the importance of clear and precise communication in the collaborative process.

Regular Cross-functional Reviews: Bring together team members from different disciplines to evaluate AI system performance and suggest improvements. They focus on technical performance metrics, clinical utility, and impact on patient care.

Iterative Development Processes: Allow for continuous refinement of prompts and AI interactions based on real-world performance and feedback from clinical users. This approach ensures that AI systems evolve to meet changing healthcare delivery needs while maintaining high accuracy and reliability standards. Ongoing contributions and a commitment to improving AI practices are crucial for the continuous advancement of healthcare AI.

Knowledge Management Systems: Capture and share insights gained through the development process, creating valuable resources for future projects and helping new team members understand the complex interplay between clinical and technical requirements.

Implementing Collaborative AI Solutions in Healthcare

In 1994, Dr. Kenneth Kizer led a groundbreaking transformation of the Veterans Health Administration (VHA), addressing widespread criticism of its poor quality and inconsistent care. His approach combined structural reorganization, cultural change, and technological advancement to create a more efficient and patient-focused system. Kizer decentralized management by establishing 22 Veterans Integrated Service Networks (VISNs), allowing local responsiveness while maintaining standardized performance metrics to ensure consistent care quality. He implemented one of healthcare's first large-scale electronic health record systems, VistA, which improved care coordination and reduced errors. Additionally, he shifted the VHA's focus from hospital-based care to patient-centered primary care, enhancing access and satisfaction. Kizer's strategy uniquely balanced clear, top-down strategic goals with bottom-up flexibility for local implementation, overcoming resistance and driving significant improvements in patient outcomes. Within five years, the VHA was recognized as a model for quality care, often outperforming private sector providers, highlighting the importance of aligning systematic planning with cultural transformation in healthcare.

Healthcare organizations must establish clear governance policies that define roles and responsibilities across disciplinary boundaries. Participants include clinical, technical, and administrative representatives, ensuring the consideration of all perspectives in decision-making. The governance framework should also establish clear protocols for handling challenges that arise during implementation and operation.

Successful healthcare AI implementation requires training programs targeted at end users. While these staff are not tasked with creating prompts for AI system development, they should understand how to develop effective prompts to obtain valid responses when using the system. Tiered training provides different levels of detail appropriate to specific roles to ensure that all staff understand the fundamental principles of healthcare AI.

Organizations that excel in healthcare AI implementation establish communities of practice that bring together end users from different disciplines to share experiences and insights. These communities provide forums for informal knowledge exchange and relationship building, complementing more formal collaborative environments.

Leadership is responsible for establishing and maintaining a collaborative culture. Effective leaders actively demonstrate commitment to cross-disciplinary collaboration and provide resources and support for cooperative initiatives. This commitment includes ensuring that reward and recognition systems encourage collaborative behavior and that career development paths recognize the value of cross-disciplinary expertise.

Evaluating Prompts

Documentation of prompt engineering practices is essential in healthcare settings, where consistency and reliability are crucial to protect patients from harm. Organizations must establish clear protocols for creating, testing, and refining prompts in developing AI tools. These protocols include mechanisms for validating prompts against clinical requirements and monitoring their effectiveness in real-world use. Successful organizations establish mechanisms for capturing and sharing lessons learned through implementation experiences, creating virtuous continuous improvement cycles.

The development of prompt libraries and best practice repositories helps organizations capture and share knowledge about practical prompt engineering approaches. These resources include technical details and insights into the collaborative processes that led to successful outcomes. Regularly reviewing and updating these resources ensures they remain relevant and valuable as technology and practices evolve.

Successful implementation is measured across multiple dimensions, including clinical outcomes, organizational effectiveness, and patient experience. Organizations must establish metrics capturing implementation and deployment's quantitative and qualitative aspects, including clinical, technical, and operational outcomes.

The challenge of effecting change in all organizations remains stubbornly tricky, yet some techniques help leaders in their efforts. My next *Bedside Consult* explores these persistent challenges and provides practical strategies for effective change management in healthcare organizations.

Bedside Consult: Turn and Face the Strange, Changes

Implementing change in a healthcare setting is a complex endeavor, with the challenges varying significantly between staff who provide direct patient care and those who do not. For those providing direct patient care, changes in processes and workflows can directly impact patients, raising the stakes of the change. Any change can lead to increased resistance, especially if staff believe the change could negatively affect patient care. Conversely, staff not working directly with patients might focus more on how the change impacts their roles or the organization.

The Challenge of Change

Changing processes and workflows in a healthcare provider organization can be challenging due to various obstacles.

Clinicians often face significant time constraints due to high patient loads and demanding schedules, making adjusting to new processes difficult. Staff not directly involved in patient care may have more flexibility to adapt to changes.

Emotional factors also play a role, with healthcare providers often having strong emotional connections to their work and patients. Changes perceived to interfere with the patient-provider relationship or the quality of care will meet strong resistance. Staff not directly involved with patients might focus more on practical considerations, such as how the change affects their workload or job responsibilities.

Regulatory and compliance considerations are another factor. Changes involving direct patient care must comply with strict regulations and standards to ensure patient safety and privacy, which can slow down and complicate the implementation of change. For staff not working directly with patients, these considerations may be less of a concern, allowing for more flexibility and speed in implementing change.

Changing processes and workflows impacting patient care require coordination among teams of professionals from different disciplines and roles. This need for interdisciplinary collaboration may be less pronounced for staff who do not work directly with patients.

Obstacles to Change

Changing processes and workflows in a healthcare provider organization can indeed be a challenging task due to a variety of obstacles. People often feel comfortable with their current ways of working and may resist change, especially if they do not understand the reasons for the change or perceive it as threatening their job security or status.

Adequate training is required to effect change. If staff members are not adequately trained in the new processes and workflows, they may be unable to adapt to the changes, leading to errors, inefficiencies, and frustration.

Without communicating the reasons for process change, staff are likely to resist or lack engagement in implementing new processes. Staff need to understand the impact of the changes on them and the organization.

Healthcare staff often work under high pressure and tight schedules, and implementing new processes and workflows can be seen as an additional burden, especially if it is perceived to increase workload or decrease efficiency. This can also lead to resistance.

Changes often require added resources, such as new software or equipment, additional staff, or an increased budget. If these resources are unavailable, it can hinder the implementation of new processes and workflows.

The organization's culture also significantly affects how change is received. If the culture does not support change or innovation, staff may be less likely to embrace new working methods. Similarly, leaders need to support the changes and model the new behaviors so that staff may be more likely to adopt the latest processes and workflows.

Steps to Foster Change

Effecting change in a healthcare organization, especially among clinical staff, requires careful planning, communication, and follow-through. Here are some best practices a healthcare manager should follow:

Clear Communication: Communicate the reasons for the change, its benefits, and how it will be implemented. Inform everyone early and often, using multiple channels of communication.

Involve staff in the Process: Involve clinical staff in the planning and implementation process. This increases buy-in, reduces resistance, and provides valuable insights to improve the change process.

Provide Adequate Training and Support: Ensure staff have the training and resources to adapt to the new processes or workflows, including formal training sessions, written guidelines, and one-on-one support.

Lead by Example: Leaders must model the new behaviors and attitudes they want to see in their staff. This behavior reinforces the change and shows support from the highest levels of the organization.

Address Concerns and Objections: Be open to feedback and ready to address concerns or objections. This helps alleviate fears, clear up misunderstandings, and build trust.

Monitor and Adjust: After implementing change, monitor its impact and be ready to make adjustments as needed to ensure that the change is effective and to minimize any negative consequences.

Celebrate Successes: Recognize and celebrate successes to build momentum, reinforce change, and boost morale.

Patient-Centered Approach: Always focus on improving patient care, keeping everyone motivated and aligned with the organization's mission.

Remember, change is a process, not an event. It takes time for people to adjust to new ways of doing things, and there may be setbacks along the way. Patience, persistence, and a positive attitude can go a long way in effecting successful change.

The successful implementation of artificial intelligence in healthcare requires more than technological sophistication—it demands the careful orchestration of people, processes, and systems. Organizations must master three critical elements: the thoughtful development of AI training prompts through clinical-technical collaboration, the establishment of robust interdisciplinary frameworks that bridge traditional silos, and the implementation of change management strategies. Healthcare leaders must remember that successful healthcare transformation is never solely about the technology—it is about empowering people to use technology effectively, building teams that can innovate continuously, and ultimately improving the quality of patient care. As healthcare organizations continue this transformation journey, maintaining this human-centered perspective is essential to realize healthcare AI's full potential.

CHAPTER 17

Workforce Transformation

In 1965, the U.S. Postal Service installed its first optical character recognition (OCR) system in a post office in Baltimore, Maryland. Workers initially resisted OCR due to fears of job loss, skepticism about the technology's reliability, and concerns that automation might devalue their skills and alter their roles within the organization. Despite this resistance, the initiative was successful through a thoughtful workforce transformation strategy. The Postal Service prioritized worker retraining to equip employees with new skills, maintained transparent communication to alleviate fears about job security, and implemented the technology gradually, allowing it to complement rather than replace existing processes.

Successful use of artificial intelligence (AI) hinges not on the technology itself but on healthcare organizations' ability to effectively manage the human aspects of change. This transformation requires a deliberate and thoughtful approach to change management that acknowledges the complexities of healthcare workflows and the vital importance of engaging all stakeholders in the process.

Healthcare organizations are confronted with distinct challenges. The stakes are notably high, as workflow changes directly impact patient care and safety while disrupting established staff routines. The workforce is a diverse mix of professionals with varying levels of technical expertise, from highly specialized clinicians to administrative staff, each with unique perspectives and concerns about the impact of AI on their jobs. The success of AI implementation depends on an organization's ability to navigate these complexities while staying true to its core mission of delivering high-quality patient care.

Healthcare workers must learn to use new technologies and adapt their established workflows and decision-making processes. This adaptation requires more than technical training; it necessitates a fundamental shift in how healthcare professionals think about using technology in their work.

Successful AI implementation begins with the recognition that every healthcare team member brings valuable insights into the implementation process. From frontline nurses who understand the practical realities of patient care to administrative staff who manage complex scheduling and billing processes, each perspective is crucial in creating more effective and sustainable AI-enabled workflows. Organizations that actively incorporate these diverse viewpoints increase the likelihood of successful implementations by making their staff feel valued and integral to the process.

Healthcare leaders are pivotal in setting the tone for AI implementation and ensuring its success. Beyond providing resources and technical support, leaders must create an environment that encourages open dialogue about changes and concerns about AI adoption. This environment requires clear communication channels, established feedback mechanisms, and demonstration of a genuine commitment to incorporate staff input into implementation decisions.

Effective Change Management

The transformation of AT&T's telephone system from manual to automatic switching in the early 20th century provides a compelling example of workforce adaptation to technological innovation. First introduced in 1919 with the installation of the Panel Switch in Omaha, Nebraska, the shift faced significant resistance from operators, who feared job displacement, and customers, who questioned the system's reliability. AT&T implemented a systematic change management approach to address these concerns, including extensive training programs to prepare workers for new roles and transparent communication to build trust in the technology. The company ensured a smoother transition and achieved widespread adoption by gradually introducing automatic switching alongside manual processes. This case demonstrates the importance of workforce retraining, clear communication, and phased implementation in successfully managing transformative technologies.

A structured approach to change management provides the foundation for successful AI implementation. While each organization's journey is unique, certain fundamental principles guide effective transformation. Organizations should create a clear vision for change that aligns with their mission and values while addressing the practical concerns of those most affected by new technologies.

Before introducing AI solutions, organizations must understand their current clinical and administrative workflows. This understanding goes beyond simple process mapping to include the nuanced ways professionals make decisions, collaborate with colleagues, and interact with patients. Each workflow has formal and informal elements developed to meet specific needs and address unusual circumstances. Documenting and analyzing these workflows provide crucial insights into where AI can add the most value and how its implementation might affect established practices.

Healthcare organizations often discover that standard workflows vary significantly across departments and among individual practitioners. While it is sometimes necessary to accommodate specific needs, organizations should carefully consider these variations when designing new AI-enabled processes. The goal is not to eliminate all variation but to understand which differences serve essential purposes and which require standardization to improve efficiency and outcomes.

Sidebar: Building a Culture of Innovation and Learning

Healthcare leaders play a crucial role in fostering a culture of innovation and learning. They balance the excitement of new possibilities with the practical realities of healthcare delivery and preventing patient harm. Leaders can inspire a culture of continuous learning and improvement by creating an environment where staff feel empowered to experiment with new approaches while maintaining their commitment to quality care, patient safety, and positive patient experiences.

Professional development is crucial in building a culture of innovation and learning. Beyond technical training, staff need ongoing opportunities to develop new skills in data interpretation, AI-assisted decision-making, and workflow optimization. These learning opportunities evolve as AI implementation is not a one-time event but a continuous journey of improvement and adaptation.

Meaningful stakeholder engagement is a critical element of successful change management. This engagement should begin early in the planning process and continue throughout implementation and go-live dates. Successful organizations create multiple channels for stakeholder input, recognizing that different groups may have different communication preferences. By stressing the importance of stakeholder engagement, organizations can foster a sense of ownership and commitment among their staff, which is crucial for the successful implementation of AI.

Clinicians must engage as true partners in the transformation process. Their expertise and understanding of patient care requirements are essential for designing effective AI-enabled workflows that produce desired outcomes and do not disrupt care delivery. It also helps build buy-in and support for change among influential leaders who can serve as champions for transformation efforts.

Administrative staff bring valuable insights into the practical aspects of healthcare operations. Their understanding of scheduling, billing, and other administrative processes can identify opportunities for AI to streamline operations, improve efficiency, and enhance relationships with patients. Including administrative perspectives ensures that new workflows are practical, sustainable, and staff and patient-friendly.

Resistance to change often stems from legitimate concerns about patient safety, quality of care, and professional autonomy. Rather than viewing resistance as an obstacle to overcome, organizations should treat it as valuable feedback that can improve implementation efforts. This approach requires creating safe spaces for staff to express concerns and for leadership to share how staff input shapes implementation decisions. By acknowledging and addressing resistance constructively, organizations foster a more positive and collaborative work environment.

Familiar sources of resistance include fears about job security, technology reliability, and worries about maintaining the human element in patient care. Organizations should address these concerns openly and honestly, providing clear information about how AI will affect different roles and demonstrating a commitment to supporting staff through the transition.

Building for the Future

In 1953, Toyota revolutionized manufacturing by introducing the *andon cord system*, a pivotal innovation in quality control that empowered workers to halt production whenever they identified a problem. Initially, this approach faced resistance from management, who feared that allowing workers such authority would disrupt productivity. However, Taiichi Ohno, the architect of Toyota's production system, championed the idea, emphasizing worker empowerment's importance in fostering a continuous improvement culture. Over time, this shift from rigid, top-down control to collaborative problem-solving became a cornerstone of Toyota's success, significantly enhancing product quality and operational efficiency. This transformation illustrates how empowering workers to engage with technology and processes leads to sustainable advancements.

Successful organizations develop capabilities and structures that support continuous improvement. This long-term perspective helps ensure that initial implementation successes translate into sustainable improvements in healthcare delivery.

Creating sustainable change requires building new capabilities and processes that can evolve as technology and healthcare needs change. Organizations must develop internal expertise in managing AI-enabled workflows while creating policies that support ongoing learning and adaptation. Transparent decision-making processes balance the need for oversight with the ability to respond quickly to emerging opportunities and challenges. Effective leaders seek feedback from all key stakeholder groups, ensuring that diverse perspectives inform healthcare AI's ongoing development and adoption.

Long-term success requires building internal expertise in managing AI-enabled applications and supporting ongoing transformation efforts. Successful organizations invest in expanding staff skill sets and creating career paths that recognize the importance of technological knowledge in delivering quality patient care. This investment reduces the dependence on external consultants while building internal capacity for continuous improvement.

Training programs help staff maintain current skills and develop new ones. Creating opportunities for staff to share knowledge and experiences builds a collective understanding of effective healthcare AI practices.

Successful organizations maintain awareness of emerging technologies and evolving care delivery models that may affect their use of AI. Organizations should establish processes for evaluating new technologies, ensuring that decisions about adoption align with organizational goals and capabilities. This evaluation considers technical feasibility and human factors, focusing on improving patient care while supporting staff effectiveness.

While organizations focus on change management and workforce transformation strategies, they must also consider the regulatory environment that ensures AI tools deliver meaningful improvements in patient care. My next *Bedside Consult* examines the role of process and outcome measures in regulating healthcare AI.

Bedside Consult: Setting the Standard—The Critical Role of Outcome-Centric Healthcare AI Regulation

As AI rapidly evolves from a futuristic vision to a tangible reality, we must prioritize patient outcomes in developing AI-driven care tools. In the *JAMA* article, "Regulate artificial intelligence in health care by prioritizing patient outcomes," Ayers et al. (2024)

underscore this view by exploring how harnessing AI can genuinely enhance healthcare delivery, ensuring that technology is a boon rather than a bane to patient care.

The authors argue for a regulatory framework anchored in outcome-centric evaluations of healthcare AI technologies. This perspective challenges traditional process-centric regulations, which, while necessary, may not sufficiently address AI's unique complexities and rapid advancements. The authors elucidate AI's potential to significantly improve patient care while emphasizing the need for empirical evidence demonstrating that AI tools lead to clinically meaningful improvements in patient outcomes.

Pitfalls of Untested AI

The authors share the results of a study of the Epic Sepsis Model (ESM) as evidence of pitfalls in using AI without proper outcomes evaluation. In that study of 2,552 hospitalized patients who developed sepsis, the ESM identified only 7% who did not already receive early treatment. Moreover, the system failed to identify 67% of patients who developed sepsis.

The authors propose an outcome-centric regulatory strategy for AI, requiring companies to demonstrate that AI tools produce clinically meaningful differences in patient outcomes before being offered to customers. Regulating healthcare AI using outcome measures presents distinct challenges compared to process measures due to AI's inherent complexities and *black-box* nature.

The rapid pace of AI development often outstrips the ability of regulatory frameworks to keep up. This fast pace delivers fewer opportunities to learn from experience using these tools, which is critical for developing process-centric regulations. The novelty and complexity of AI applications make it challenging to establish standardized outcome measures universally applicable across different technologies, diseases, and patient populations.

Measuring Outcomes

Outcome measures also require empirical evidence demonstrating that AI applications lead to a net clinically meaningful improvement in patient outcomes compared to existing standards of care or placebo. This necessitates rigorous, long-term studies, such as randomized clinical trials, to establish the efficacy and safety of AI tools. Such studies are time-consuming and resource-intensive and may need to be continuously updated to account for AI advancements, retraining of models on different data sets, and changes in clinical practice.

Furthermore, outcome-centric regulation requires the establishment of clear, measurable endpoints that accurately reflect improvements in patient health. These endpoints must be clinically meaningful, directly tied to patient well-being, and sensitive enough to capture the effects of AI interventions. The complexity of healthcare and the variability in patient responses add layers of difficulty in defining and measuring these outcomes.

In addition, outcome measures must consider AI's broader impact on the healthcare ecosystem, including effects on clinical staff workload, patient-clinician interactions, and ethical dilemmas. These factors are less tangible than process measures and require a holistic evaluation of AI technologies' integration into healthcare workflows.

As the authors point out, process-centric regulations, while easier to define and enforce, may not adequately prevent harm or ensure improvements in patient outcomes when applied to AI. Process measures focus on the steps taken to develop and deploy AI technologies rather than on their actual impact on patient health.

The advent of electronic health records has provided a wealth of data that researchers can leverage to test the impact and outcomes of various AI clinical tools. Organizations like the Mayo Clinic are at the forefront of building comprehensive databases that can be a bedrock for evaluating AI technologies in clinical settings.

These databases offer a unique opportunity to rigorously assess the effectiveness of AI applications in improving patient outcomes, thereby ensuring that the integration of AI in healthcare is both evidence-based and outcome-driven.

Need for Regulating Agency

One must recognize AI's power to revolutionize patient care through predictive analytics, personalized treatment plans, and advanced diagnostic tools. Yet, the allure of these advancements should not overshadow the necessity for these technologies to demonstrate a tangible, positive impact on patient outcomes. It is here that the Agency for Healthcare Research and Quality (AHRQ), a component of the US Department of Health and Human Services (DHSS), can play a pivotal role in setting the standards for AI use in healthcare.

AHRQ's mission centers on producing evidence to make health care safer, higher quality, more accessible, equitable, and affordable, and to work within the DHSS and with other partners to ensure that the evidence is understood and used. Through research, data, and analytics, AHRQ informs health policy and practice, aiming to improve the outcomes and quality of healthcare services. The agency's work encompasses many healthcare issues, including patient safety, healthcare improvement, health information technology, and access to healthcare services. By generating rigorous and relevant evidence, AHRQ supports healthcare professionals and policymakers in making informed decisions that improve healthcare delivery and patient outcomes. AHRQ possesses the skilled staff to undertake AI evaluation and propose regulations.

Beyond Outcomes

The integration of AI in healthcare extends beyond patient outcomes. Researchers must consider the impact of AI tools on clinical staff. Effective deployment of AI requires supporting clinical staff, reducing their workload, and minimizing burnout without introducing ethical dilemmas or compromising their *duty of care* responsibilities. This dual focus—on both patient outcomes and the well-being of clinical staff—is crucial for the moral and effective implementation of AI in healthcare.

Regulating AI in healthcare using outcome measures is more challenging than using process measures due to the need for empirical evidence of clinical benefit, the complexities of defining and measuring meaningful patient outcomes, and the rapid evolution of AI technologies. These challenges necessitate a nuanced, flexible, and patient-centered approach to regulation that can adapt to the fast-paced advancements in AI, ensuring that these technologies truly enhance patient care.

Implementing artificial intelligence in healthcare is a critical inflection point in medicine's digital transformation. Success requires organizations to balance technological sophistication with human factors—engaging stakeholders, building sustainable processes, and focusing on patient care. As healthcare organizations progress in their AI journeys, they must remember that lasting transformation comes not through technology alone but through careful attention to the human elements of change. Healthcare organizations can harness AI's potential while preserving their core mission of delivering high-quality, patient-centered care by building robust strategies for change management, stakeholder engagement, and governance.

CHAPTER 18

The Patient-Physician Journey to 2050

In 1959, Harold Hopkins, a physicist, developed a break-through technology that would later revolutionize surgery: the rod-lens optical system. This system significantly enhanced the clarity and brightness of images transmitted through an *endoscope*, a device used to view inside the body. Unlike previous fiber-optic technologies, the rod-lens system reduced light loss and distortion, making seeing internal structures with unprecedented detail possible. In 1960, Karl Storz, a medical instrument manufacturer, collaborated with Hopkins to refine and produce these advanced endoscopes for medical use.

Fast-forward to the 1980s, when a convergence of technologies propelled laparoscopic surgery into mainstream use. The development of high-resolution miniature video cameras, first introduced in 1981, allowed surgeons to project live images from inside the body onto monitors. This innovation transformed the practice by enabling surgeons to perform procedures with enhanced visualization. In 1987, Dr. Philippe Mouret performed the first laparoscopic chole-cystectomy in Lyon, France. This event marked the true beginning of modern laparoscopic surgery.

The widespread adoption of laparoscopic techniques in the 1990s required a significant transformation in healthcare delivery. Surgeons had to abandon the surgical techniques they had perfected and adopt entirely new operating methods, relying on video monitors and specialized instruments rather than direct visualization. Operating room staff, including nurses and anesthesiologists, adapted to new workflows, equipment, and teamwork dynamics. Initially, many clinicians resisted this change, citing concerns over patient safety, the technical challenges of using laparoscopic equipment, and the disruption to traditional methods.

Despite these challenges, the benefits of laparoscopic surgery are undeniable. Compared to open surgery, patients experience shorter recovery times, reduced post-operative pain, and fewer complications. Over time, the medical community embraced laparoscopic techniques, and their application expanded to include complex procedures such as appendectomies, hysterectomies, and even cardiac surgery.

The adoption of laparoscopic surgery did not just improve healthcare delivery—it also enhanced the roles of clinicians. Surgeons became skilled in advanced technology, elevating their expertise while operating room teams developed greater collaboration and efficiency. The transformation demonstrated how embracing new tools and methods could lead to better patient outcomes, enhanced professional satisfaction, and a more efficient healthcare system.

The journey of laparoscopic surgery—from the invention of the rod-lens system in 1959 to its widespread adoption in the 1990s—illustrates the profound impact of technological innovation on medicine. It serves as a reminder that while change can be challenging, it ultimately empowers clinicians and benefits patients when guided by vision, training, and willingness to adapt. This same spirit of innovation underpins the opportunities we face today with artificial intelligence (AI) in healthcare. By embracing these technologies, we can once again transform how we deliver care, improving outcomes for all.

Our Role

As we conclude our journey through healthcare AI, I am optimistic about the future we can create together. Throughout these pages, we explored the technical foundations of AI in healthcare and the profound ways these technologies can enhance our ability to serve patients, support healthcare professionals, and strengthen our healthcare systems. The path ahead is challenging and inspiring—it demands our careful attention, ethical commitment, and unwavering focus on improving human lives.

The healthcare AI revolution we examined is not primarily about technology—it is about people. It is about giving clinicians more time to connect meaningfully with patients by reducing the administrative burden. It is about empowering nurses with predictive insights that help them deliver more proactive care. It is about providing administrative staff with tools that make their work more efficient and meaningful. Most importantly, it is about creating a healthcare system that better serves all members of our society, including those in traditionally underserved communities.

Our exploration began with understanding AI's foundations in healthcare, examining how these technologies can augment clinical expertise while preserving clinician autonomy. We then delved into strategic approaches for implementation, considering everything from research methods to economic implications. Finally, we tackled the critical challenges of leading this transformation—building trust, managing change, and ensuring the primacy of patient safety.

The knowledge you gained provides a comprehensive framework for implementing AI in ways that enhance rather than disrupt healthcare delivery. You understand now that successful AI implementation requires more than technical expertise—it demands thoughtful leadership, effective change management, and an unwavering commitment to ethical principles. You learned to build teams that bridge clinical excellence and technological innovation, establish robust validation protocols, and create the trust necessary for successful adoption.

As you progress with your AI initiatives, remember that this transformation is a continuing patient-physician journey supported by all who impact healthcare delivery. Technology will continue to evolve, but the fundamental principles we explored remain constant: maintain focus on patient benefit, ensure ethical implementation, support your workforce through change, and always strive to improve healthcare delivery. Success requires balancing innovation with responsibility, efficiency with safety, and technological capabilities with human judgment.

I encourage you to approach this transformation with both ambition and humility. Be ambitious in your vision for how AI can improve healthcare delivery but humble in recognizing the complexity of implementation and the paramount importance of patient safety. Embrace these technologies' potential while maintaining rigorous validation and monitoring standards. Most importantly, never lose sight of the human element in healthcare—AI should enhance, not replace, the compassion and judgment that define excellent patient care.

The future of healthcare lies not in choosing between human expertise and artificial intelligence but in thoughtfully combining both to create something greater than either alone. When implemented wisely, AI can help us build a healthcare system that is more proactive, personalized, and equitable. It can help us shift from episodic to preventive care, from standardized to personalized treatments, and from fragmented to integrated healthcare delivery.

As you leave these pages, I hope you feel equipped and inspired to lead this transformation in your organization. The frameworks, strategies, and insights we explored provide a roadmap for success, but the journey ahead requires your leadership and vision.

Remember that every AI implementation decision impacts not just operational efficiency but people's lives—your patients, your staff, and your community.

The technology is powerful, but its true value lies in how we use it to reshape healthcare delivery for society's benefit. The future of healthcare is not something that happens to us—it is something we create together, one thoughtful decision at a time. Let us embrace this opportunity with wisdom, responsibility, and unwavering commitment. While the journey ahead is complex, the potential rewards—for our patients, our healthcare workforce, and our society—make it profoundly worthwhile.

Afterword

Throughout this book, we explored how artificial intelligence can transform healthcare, enhancing our ability to diagnose, treat, and care for patients. The potential benefits are enormous: more accurate diagnoses, personalized treatments, streamlined operations, and improved patient outcomes. Yet, as we embrace these advances, we must also confront a broader challenge that AI presents to society—its potential to blur the line between truth and fiction.

> **"You submit to tyranny when you renounce the difference between what you want to hear and what is actually the case."**
>
> —Snyder, T. (2017). *On tyranny: Twenty lessons from the twentieth century* (p. 66) Tim Duggan Books

This warning takes on new urgency in our age of artificial intelligence. As we enter an era where AI can generate increasingly convincing deepfakes and fabricated audio, video, and written content, the very foundation of human trust is threatened. The same technologies that promise to enhance healthcare also possess the capability to erode the bedrock of democratic society—our ability to distinguish fact from fiction.

The essence of human society rests upon our initial inclination to trust one another. Yet when we can no longer trust our eyes and ears, when any image, voice, or article might be an AI fabrication, the bonds that hold our communities together begin to fray. This technological capability to manipulate reality undermines our democratic institutions and the fundamental bonds of trust between people that make civil society possible.

In this context, journalists who maintain rigorous standards of truth-telling and fact-checking serve as essential guardians against both human and AI-generated deception. Their work—investigating, verifying, and reporting truth—serves as humanity's immune system against the virulent spread of misinformation, whether crafted by authoritarian regimes or artificial intelligence. From newsrooms to war zones, these dedicated professionals risk their freedom and often their lives to ensure that citizens can make informed decisions about their governance and their future.

The lessons of history, particularly the dark descent of the 1930s, remind us that democracy's strength lies not in its inevitability but in its careful maintenance. Today, as AI adds new weapons to the arsenal of potential manipulation and control, the role of honest journalists becomes even more crucial. As the United States—the world's first and longest-lasting modern democracy—enshrined in its *Declaration of Independence*, our rights to *life, liberty, and the pursuit of happiness* require constant vigilance and protection.

The challenge before us is to remain vigilant against AI's potential harms while harnessing its remarkable benefits for human advancement. This delicate balance requires trusted voices who can help us navigate between innovation and risk, between progress and preservation of human values. Journalists who earn and maintain our trust serve as a bulwark against those who would use AI to control our lives and diminish our freedoms, whether they be authoritarian regimes or other malicious actors.

Just as we have seen throughout this book, the promise of AI in healthcare can only be realized in a society where truth is valued, where facts matter, and where the free exchange of ideas is protected. The journalists who defend these principles, often at terrible personal cost, safeguard not just information but the possibility of human advancement in an age where the line between reality and artificial creation grows increasingly blurred.

Yet, even as we acknowledge these challenges, we can remain hopeful about our future. The same human spirit that drives journalists to seek truth despite danger and opposition also drives healthcare professionals, researchers, and innovators to push the boundaries of what is possible in medicine. When we combine human wisdom with technological advancement, when we balance innovation with integrity, and when we remain committed to truth and transparency, we can ensure that AI becomes a force for good in healthcare and throughout society.

The future belongs not to those who would use technology to deceive and control but to those who harness it with compassion and vision to serve humanity's highest aspirations. In this endeavor, we honor both the journalists who safeguard truth and the healthcare pioneers who work tirelessly to transform that truth into better lives for all. As we close this exploration of artificial intelligence in healthcare, let us remember that every technological advance must be guided by our highest human values—the pursuit of truth, the protection of dignity, and the preservation of freedom.

Glossary

Acute Coronary Syndrome (ACS): A group of clinical conditions caused by sudden, reduced blood flow to the heart, leading to symptoms such as chest pain, shortness of breath, and other signs of cardiac ischemia. ACS encompasses three primary conditions: unstable angina, non-ST-elevation myocardial infarction (NSTEMI), and ST-elevation myocardial infarction (STEMI). Prompt diagnosis and treatment of ACS are critical to restore blood flow and prevent irreversible heart muscle damage.

Acute Respiratory Distress Syndrome (ARDS): A severe lung condition characterized by the rapid onset of widespread inflammation and fluid buildup in the lungs. This condition leads to difficulty breathing and low blood oxygen levels. ARDS often results from conditions such as sepsis, trauma, or pneumonia and requires immediate medical intervention.

Algorithmovigilance: A system for monitoring and addressing risks associated with machine learning and AI algorithms, ensuring accuracy, fairness, and safety in healthcare applications. Algorithmovigilance promotes reliable and ethical AI decision-making while safeguarding patient safety and data integrity.

Ambulatory Glucose Profile (AGP): A standardized graphical representation of glucose levels in individuals using continuous glucose monitoring systems. It visualizes glucose trends over several days, allowing for a better understanding of glycemic patterns, variability, and areas for improvement in diabetes management.

Andon Cord: A visual or physical signaling mechanism used in manufacturing or production environments to indicate a problem in the workflow or a need for assistance. Originally popularized in Toyota's lean manufacturing system, the andon cord allows workers to halt production when an issue is identified, enabling immediate attention and resolution. This tool promotes quality control, empowers employees to address problems proactively, and minimizes defects by ensuring issues are resolved before production continues. In modern settings, the andon cord may be a literal cord, a button, or a digital alert system.

Application Programming Interface (API): A set of protocols, tools, and definitions that allow software applications to communicate with one another. APIs integrate systems, enabling seamless data exchange and functionality within and between healthcare applications.

Area Under the Receiver Operating Characteristic Curve (AUROC): A statistical measure used to evaluate the performance of binary classification models. It plots the true positive rate against the false positive rate at various threshold levels, with the area under the curve indicating model accuracy. A value closer to 1.0 signifies higher diagnostic accuracy.

Artificial Intelligence (AI): A field of computer science focused on creating systems that perform tasks typically requiring human intelligence, such as problem-solving, pattern recognition, learning, and decision-making. AI can assist in diagnosing diseases, predicting patient outcomes, and automating administrative tasks.

Artificial Intelligence Act (AIA): A proposed European Union regulation to ensure the ethical and safe development of artificial intelligence (AI). The AIA classifies AI systems into unacceptable, high, and lower-risk categories, requiring stricter oversight for high-risk applications like healthcare AI while fostering innovation for lower-risk uses.

Attention Mechanism: A machine learning technique that directs deep learning models to prioritize (or attend to) the most relevant parts of input data. Innovation in attention mechanisms enabled the transformer architecture to yield the modern large language models (LLMs) that power popular applications like ChatGPT.

Augmented Reality (AR): A technology that overlays digital information, such as images, sounds, or text, onto the real-world environment. AR can assist in surgical procedures, medical education, and patient engagement by providing visual enhancements and real-time data.

Automated Insulin Delivery (AID): An advanced diabetes management system that integrates a continuous glucose monitor and an insulin pump to automate insulin delivery. The system adjusts insulin doses based on real-time glucose readings, reducing the risk of hypoglycemia and hyperglycemia.

Aviation Safety Reporting System (ASRS): A voluntary, confidential reporting system administered by NASA for the Federal Aviation Administration (FAA). It collects and analyzes aviation-related safety reports from pilots, controllers, and other personnel to identify and address safety issues, improving overall aviation safety.

Body Mass Index (BMI): A numerical value calculated from an individual's weight and height, used to assess body fatness and categorize individuals into weight categories such as underweight, normal weight, overweight, and obese. BMI is a simple, widely used tool in public health for screening and monitoring weight-related health risks.

Business Associate Agreement (BAA): A legally binding agreement between a healthcare provider and a business associate that outlines how protected health information (PHI) is used, disclosed, and protected by the Health Insurance Portability and Accountability Act (HIPAA) regulations. The BAA ensures that both parties comply with HIPAA privacy and security standards.

Causal Machine Learning: A branch of machine learning focused on identifying and leveraging cause-and-effect relationships within data. Unlike traditional machine learning, which emphasizes correlation, causal machine learning uses techniques like causal inference and structural modeling to determine how changes in one variable affect others. Healthcare researchers use it to understand treatment effects, predict patient outcomes under different interventions, and improve decision-making by distinguishing causation from mere association.

CE Marking: A certification indicating that a product meets safety, health, and environmental protection standards for sale in the European Economic Area (EEA). **CE** marking applies to various products, including medical devices, ensuring compliance with regulatory requirements.

Center for Disease Control and Prevention: A U.S. federal government agency whose mission is to protect public health by preventing and controlling disease, injury, and disability. The CDC promotes healthy behaviors and safe, healthy environments. It keeps track of health trends, tries to find the cause of health problems and disease outbreaks, and responds to new public health threats. The CDC works with state health departments and other organizations throughout the country and the world to help prevent and control disease.

Centers for Medicare & Medicaid Services (CMS): A federal agency within the U.S. Department of Health and Human Services responsible for administering the nation's major healthcare programs, including Medicare, Medicaid, the Children's Health Insurance Program (CHIP), and the Health Insurance Marketplace. CMS oversees regulations, payment systems, and quality standards to ensure access to healthcare for millions of Americans.

Centers for Medicare & Medicaid Services Hierarchical Condition Category (CMS-HCC): A risk adjustment model used by CMS to determine payments for Medicare Advantage plans and certain other programs. The model assigns a risk score to each enrollee based on their demographic characteristics and health conditions, enabling CMS to predict healthcare costs and allocate appropriate resources for patients with varying levels of health complexity.

Chemical Cross-Linking Mass Spectrometry (CXMS): A technique to analyze proteins' three-dimensional structure and interactions. CXMS involves chemically cross-linking proteins at specific sites and using mass spectrometry to identify cross-linked peptides. This method provides insights into protein conformations, interactions, and structural changes, contributing to studying protein complexes and drug design.

Chronic Obstructive Pulmonary Disease (COPD): A group of progressive lung diseases, including emphysema and chronic bronchitis, that cause chronic airway obstruction and breathing difficulties. COPD is often linked to long-term exposure to irritants like cigarette smoke and is managed with medication, lifestyle changes, and pulmonary rehabilitation.

Clinical Decision Support (CDS): A health information technology system that provides clinicians, staff, and patients with intelligently filtered information at appropriate times to enhance health and healthcare decision-making. CDS tools include alerts, reminders, clinical guidelines, and diagnostic support systems to improve care quality and safety.

Clinical Practice Guidelines (CPG): Recommendations on diagnosing and treating a medical condition based on medical evidence and professional expertise. They are written for doctors, nurses, and other health care professionals.

Complete Blood Count (CBC): A standard blood test that evaluates overall health and detects various disorders by measuring several components of blood, including red blood cells, white blood cells, hemoglobin, hematocrit, and platelets. A CBC helps diagnose anemia, infections, and other hematologic abnormalities.

Computed Tomography (CT): An imaging technique that uses X-rays and computer processing to create detailed cross-sectional images of the body. CT scans are widely used in diagnostic medicine to visualize internal organs, bones, soft tissues, and blood vessels, aiding in diagnosing and managing various medical conditions.

Computer Vision: A field of artificial intelligence that enables computers to interpret, analyze, and extract meaningful information from visual data such as images and videos.

Congestive Heart Failure (CHF): A chronic, progressive condition in which the heart muscle is unable to pump blood effectively, leading to insufficient blood flow to meet the body's needs. Symptoms include shortness of breath, fatigue, and fluid retention. CHF is managed through lifestyle changes, medication, and, in some cases, surgical interventions.

Continuous Glucose Monitoring (CGM): A real-time tracking of glucose levels using a sensor inserted under the skin that measures interstitial glucose levels continuously. CGM systems provide trends, patterns, and alerts, helping people with diabetes make informed diet, activity, and insulin-dosing decisions.

Convolutional Neural Network (CNN): A class of deep learning algorithms primarily used for image recognition, classification, and analysis. CNNs automatically learn to identify spatial patterns in data through multiple layers of convolutional filters, making them effective for medical image analysis, visual recognition, and natural language processing.

COVID-19 (Coronavirus Disease 2019): An infectious disease caused by the severe acute respiratory syndrome coronavirus 2 (SARS-CoV-2). It emerged in late 2019 and led to a global pandemic. Symptoms range from mild respiratory issues to severe pneumonia, and in some cases, it can lead to complications such as acute respiratory distress syndrome (ARDS) and multi-organ failure. The disease was managed through public health measures, vaccinations, and treatments.

Critical Assessment of Protein Structure Prediction (CASP): A biennial scientific competition in which researchers evaluate the accuracy of computational methods for predicting protein structures. CASP serves as a benchmark for assessing progress and identifying the strengths and limitations of protein structure prediction techniques.

Cryo-electron Microscopy (Cryo-EM): A powerful imaging technique that uses a beam of electrons to visualize biological molecules at near-atomic resolution. Cryo-EM samples are rapidly frozen to preserve their natural structure, allowing researchers to study proteins, viruses, and other macromolecules in their native state without crystallization. This method has become crucial in structural biology and drug discovery.

Dark Data: A term often used in data analytics, refers to information assets that organizations collect, process, and store during regular business activities but are not used for other operational purposes.

Deep Learning: A subset of machine learning that utilizes neural networks with multiple layers to automatically learn complex patterns and features from large datasets. Deep learning is particularly effective for tasks such as image and speech recognition, natural language processing, and predictive analytics.

Differential Privacy (DP): A mathematically rigorous framework for releasing statistical information about datasets while protecting the privacy of individual data subjects. It enables a data holder to share aggregate patterns of the group while limiting the information leaked about specific individuals.

Digital Imaging and Communications in Medicine (DICOM): A standard for storing, transmitting, and sharing medical images and related data. DICOM enables the interoperability of medical imaging devices such as X-rays, CT scans, and MRIs, ensuring that images and data can be accessed and used by various healthcare providers and systems.

Dragon Ambient eXperience (DAX): A clinical documentation solution developed by Nuance that uses artificial intelligence (AI) to capture and document patient-physician conversations in real time. DAX converts spoken interactions into structured clinical notes that integrate directly into electronic health records, allowing clinicians to focus on patient care while reducing administrative workload.

Edge Computing: A distributed computing model that brings computation and data storage closer to the data sources. More broadly, it refers to any design that pushes computation physically closer to a user to reduce the latency compared to when an application runs on a centralized data center.

Electronic Health Record (EHR): A digital version of a patient's paper chart that contains comprehensive health information, including medical history, diagnoses, medications, treatment plans, immunization dates, allergies, radiology images, and laboratory test results. EHRs facilitate information sharing among healthcare providers, improving care coordination and patient safety.

Emergency Department (ED): A medical treatment facility that cares for patients with acute illnesses or injuries requiring immediate medical attention. The ED, commonly called the emergency room (ER), is equipped to provide rapid diagnosis, stabilization, and treatment of critical conditions.

Epidemic Intelligence Service (EIS): A 2-year postgraduate program run by the Centers for Disease Control and Prevention (CDC). Often called the CDC's *disease detectives*, EIS officers are trained public health professionals investigating and rsponding to disease outbreaks, natural disasters, and other public health emergencies.

European Molecular Biology Laboratory–European Bioinformatics Institute (EMBL-EBI): A global bioinformatics research and data services leader. EMBL-EBI is part of the European Molecular Biology Laboratory. It provides freely available data, tools, and resources for the study of molecular biology, supporting research in genomics, proteomics, and systems biology.

Explainable Artificial Intelligence (XAI): A set of techniques and methodologies aimed at making the decision-making processes of AI models transparent, understandable, and interpretable to humans. XAI is essential for ensuring trust, accountability, and regulatory compliance in healthcare, where understanding the reasoning behind AI-driven decisions is critical.

Fast Healthcare Interoperability Resources (FHIR): A standard developed by Health Level Seven International (HL7) for exchanging healthcare information electronically. FHIR defines a set of resources and interfaces for representing and sharing clinical data, enabling interoperability between different healthcare systems and improving data accessibility for healthcare providers and patients.

Feature Engineering: A preprocessing step in supervised machine learning and statistical modeling that transforms raw data into a more effective set of inputs. Each input comprises several attributes, known as features.

Feature Importance Analysis: is a technique in machine learning that determines the relative significance of each input variable (feature) in predicting an outcome, essentially identifying which features have the most impact on a model's predictions, allowing for better model interpretation and understanding of the data driving the results.

Federal Trade Commission (FTC): An independent agency of the U.S. government tasked with protecting consumers and ensuring a fair marketplace by preventing anticompetitive, deceptive, and unfair business practices. The FTC enforces regulations on health-related advertising, data privacy, and competition within the healthcare industry.

Food and Drug Administration (FDA): A U.S. federal agency within the Department of Health and Human Services responsible for protecting public health by regulating the safety, efficacy, and security of human and veterinary drugs, biological products, medical devices, food, cosmetics, and tobacco products. The FDA also oversees clinical trials and approves new treatments and medical devices for use in healthcare.

G Protein-Coupled Receptor (GPCR): A large family of cell surface receptors that play a crucial role in transmitting signals from outside the cell to the inside, influencing various physiological processes such as hormone response, neurotransmission, and immune function. GPCRs are a major target for drug development, as they are involved in many diseases and therapeutic pathways.

General Data Protection Regulation (GDPR): A European Union law that regulates the collection, processing, and storage of personal data, ensuring privacy and data security for EU residents. GDPR applies to organizations worldwide that handle EU citizens' data, including healthcare providers and tech companies.

Generative Adversarial Network (GAN): A class of machine learning models composed of two neural networks—the generator and the discriminator—that produce new, synthetic data. GANs are used for applications such as image generation, data augmentation, and simulation of realistic data for training models. The generator creates data samples, while the discriminator evaluates their authenticity, improving the quality of generated data over time.

Generative Pre-trained Transformer (GPT): A type of large language model based on the transformer architecture, designed to generate human-like text by predicting the next word in a sequence. GPT models are pre-trained on vast amounts of text, image, video, and audio data and fine-tuned for specific tasks, making them highly effective for applications like text generation, summarization, and question-answering.

Gradient Boosting: A machine learning technique that gives a prediction model in the form of an ensemble of weak prediction models, i.e., models that make very few assumptions about the data, typically simple decision trees. In healthcare, it is used for risk assessment and disease prediction tasks.

Graphics Processing Unit (GPU): A specialized electronic circuit designed to accelerate the rendering of images and videos by performing parallel processing tasks. GPUs are essential for high-performance computing applications, including deep learning, scientific research, and medical imaging, due to their ability to handle large-scale computations efficiently.

Gross Domestic Product (GDP): A monetary measure representing the total value of all goods and services produced within a country's borders over a specified period, typically a year. GDP is a key indicator of a nation's economic health and is used to assess economic growth and development.

Hardware Security Module (HSM): A physical computing device that safeguards and manages secrets (most importantly digital keys) and performs encryption and decryption functions for digital signatures, strong authentication, and other cryptographic functions. These modules traditionally come as a plug-in card or an external device that attaches directly to a computer or network server. A hardware security module contains one or more secure cryptoprocessor chips.

Health and Human Services (HHS): The U.S. government agency responsible for protecting the health of all Americans and providing essential human services. HHS oversees various healthcare programs, including Medicare, Medicaid, and public health initiatives, and enforces regulations like HIPAA to ensure patient privacy and healthcare quality.

Health Information Exchange (HIE): The electronic sharing of health-related information between different healthcare organizations to facilitate coordinated care, reduce duplication, and improve healthcare outcomes. HIEs enable providers to access and exchange patient data securely and in real time.

Health Information Technology (HIT): Using technology, such as electronic health records, telehealth, and health information exchanges, to store, retrieve, and share health information. HIT aims to improve healthcare quality, safety, and efficiency through better data management and communication.

Health Insurance Portability and Accountability Act (HIPAA): A U.S. federal law enacted in 1996 that establishes national standards for protecting sensitive patient health information. HIPAA includes provisions for data privacy, security, and the safe exchange of health information between healthcare providers, insurers, and other entities.

Health Technology Assessment (HTA): A systematic evaluation of the properties, effects, and impact of healthcare technology, including medical devices, drugs, and procedures. HTA considers clinical efficacy, safety, cost-effectiveness, and social and ethical implications to inform decision-making and healthcare policy.

Heat Map: A data visualization technique that uses color gradients to represent the magnitude of values across a dataset. Heat maps highlight areas of interest in medical images, display patient health metrics, or visualize patterns such as disease prevalence or treatment effectiveness.

Hemoglobin A1c (HbA1c): A blood test that measures the average blood glucose levels over the past two to three months by assessing the percentage of hemoglobin chemically linked to glucose. HbA1c is used to diagnose and monitor diabetes and assess long-term blood glucose control in individuals with diabetes.

HITRUST Certification: A standardized approach to managing and protecting the sensitive information found within the healthcare industry. This comprehensive approach reduces the risk of data breaches and ensures your organization complies with the required regulations.

Homomorphic Encryption: A cryptographic method enabling computations on encrypted data without decryption, preserving privacy. It is especially useful for analyzing sensitive healthcare data, though it requires substantial computational resources.

Human-in-the-loop (HITL): A collaborative approach that integrates human input and expertise into the lifecycle of machine learning and artificial intelligence systems. In healthcare, HITL is used to validate model outputs in diagnosis or treatment planning.

Industrial Internet of Things (IIoT): A subset of the Internet of Things that integrates connected devices, sensors, and data analytics into industrial processes to improve efficiency, productivity, and safety. IIoT is used in manufacturing, supply chain management, and other industrial settings to enable real-time monitoring, predictive maintenance, and process optimization.

Inflation Reduction Act: A U.S. federal law enacted in 2022 that aims to reduce inflation by lowering prescription drug prices, investing in clean energy, and increasing tax enforcement. The act includes measures to reduce healthcare costs by capping drug prices and promoting healthcare access.

Intelligent Tutoring System (ITS): A computer-based learning system that uses artificial intelligence to provide personalized instruction and student feedback. ITS adapts to individual learning needs by analyzing student performance, identifying areas for improvement, and offering customized learning pathways.

Intensive Care Unit (ICU): A specialized hospital unit that provides intensive monitoring and treatment for patients with severe or life-threatening illnesses and injuries. ICUs are equipped with advanced medical technology and staffed by specialized healthcare professionals to deliver critical care.

Internet of Medical Things (IoMT): A subset of the Internet of Things (IoT) that refers to connected medical devices and applications used for patient monitoring, diagnosis, and treatment. IoMT enables real-time health data collection and analysis, facilitating remote patient management and personalized care.

Internet of Things (IoT): A network of interconnected devices, sensors, and systems that communicate and share data over the internet. IoT enables automation, monitoring, and control of devices and systems in various settings, including healthcare, smart homes, and industrial environments.

Key Performance Indicator (KPI): A measurable value used to evaluate the performance and success of an organization, department, or individual in achieving specific objectives.

Large Language Model (LLM): An AI model trained on vast amounts of text data to understand and generate human-like language. Examples include Claude, GPT-4, and Gemini, which are widely used in text generation, translation, and conversational AI applications.

Local Interpretable Model-agnostic Explanations (LIME): A method for explaining machine learning predictions by approximating them with simpler models locally around specific instances. LIME is used in healthcare to make AI outputs interpretable for clinical decision-making.

Machine Learning (ML): A subset of artificial intelligence that involves training algorithms on data to identify patterns and make predictions or decisions without explicit programming. ML is used in various applications, including medical diagnosis, image recognition, and predictive analytics.

Magnetic Resonance Imaging (MRI): A non-invasive imaging technique that uses strong magnetic fields and radio waves to create detailed images of the body's internal structures. MRI helps diagnose and monitor various conditions, particularly those affecting soft tissues, such as the brain, spinal cord, and joints.

m-Health (Mobile Health): Using mobile devices, such as smartphones and tablets, and wearable technology to support healthcare practices, monitor health conditions, and promote wellness. m-Health includes mobile applications for tracking fitness, managing chronic conditions, enabling telehealth services, and enhancing accessibility and patient engagement.

Milliman Advanced Risk Adjusters (MARA): A predictive modeling tool used to assess risk and predict future healthcare costs based on patient data, including demographic information, diagnoses, and claims history. MARA is used by health plans, providers, and employers to identify high-risk individuals and manage healthcare resources effectively.

Model Inversion Attack: A type of AI attack during which an attacker tries to infer personal information about a data subject by exploiting the outputs of a machine learning model.

Multimodal AI: A type of artificial intelligence that processes and integrates data from multiple modalities, such as text, images, audio, and structured data, to generate more comprehensive insights and predictions. Multimodal AI combines data sources like medical images, clinical notes, and lab results to enhance diagnostic accuracy and decision-making.

Multimodal Fusion: Combining information from multiple modalities to enhance understanding or analysis of a specific phenomenon or problem. It integrates data from different sources, such as text, images, audio, video, and sensor readings, to better represent the underlying information.

Multiple Daily Injections (MDI): A method of insulin therapy used to manage blood glucose levels in individuals with diabetes. MDI typically involves administering rapid-acting insulin before meals and long-acting insulin once or twice daily to maintain basal insulin levels, providing flexibility in insulin dosing.

Multiple Sequence Alignment (MSA): A bioinformatics technique used to align three or more biological sequences, such as DNA, RNA, or proteins, to identify regions of similarity that may indicate functional, structural, or evolutionary relationships. MSA is essential for phylogenetic analysis, protein structure prediction, and gene annotation.

Multi-tenant Architecture: A software architecture where a single instance serves multiple tenants or groups of users while maintaining data separation and security. Multi-tenancy improves resource efficiency and scalability compared to systems with separate instances for each tenant.

Natural Language Processing (NLP): A field of artificial intelligence that focuses on enabling machines to understand, interpret, and generate human language. NLP is used for clinical documentation, speech recognition, and analyzing unstructured medical data to gain insights and support decision-making.

Nuclear Magnetic Resonance (NMR): A non-invasive imaging technique that uses magnetic fields and radio waves to study the structure and dynamics of molecules at the atomic level. NMR is widely used in chemistry and biochemistry to analyze the composition of substances and investigate protein structures.

Nuclear Pore Complex (NPC): A large protein complex that spans the nuclear envelope, regulating the transport of molecules such as RNA and proteins between the nucleus and the cytoplasm. The NPC is critical for maintaining cellular function and genome stability by controlling the flow of genetic information.

Office for Civil Rights (OCR): A division of the U.S. Department of Health and Human Services (HHS) responsible for enforcing civil rights and health information privacy laws, including the Health Insurance Portability and Accountability Act. OCR ensures that healthcare providers and organizations comply with regulations protecting patient privacy and preventing discrimination.

Patient-Generated Health Data (PGHD): Health-related data created, recorded, or gathered by patients, caregivers, or health-tracking devices to address a health concern. PGHD includes data on symptoms, lifestyle behaviors, and health history, which clinicians can share with healthcare providers to support treatment plans and clinical decision-making.

Personally Identifiable Information (PII): Information that can be used to identify an individual, such as name, social security number, address, email, or phone number. Protecting PII is essential to maintaining patient confidentiality and complying with privacy regulations such as HIPAA and GDPR. Protected health information is a subset of PII.

Picture Archiving and Communication System (PACS): A medical imaging technology used for storing, retrieving, presenting, and sharing images produced by different imaging modalities such as X-rays, CT scans, and MRIs. PACS eliminates the need for physical film storage, enabling efficient digital management and remote access to images.

Point-of-care Ultrasound (POCUS): A portable ultrasound imaging technique used at the patient's bedside to assess and diagnose medical conditions quickly. It is also used in emergency and critical care settings to evaluate symptoms, guide procedures, and monitor treatment responses in real time.

Positron Emission Tomography (PET): A nuclear imaging technique that uses a small amount of radioactive material to visualize and measure metabolic processes in the body. PET scans often detect cancer, evaluate brain function, and monitor heart conditions by producing detailed images of tissue and organ function.

Post-Traumatic Stress Disorder (PTSD): A mental health condition triggered by experiencing or witnessing a traumatic event. Symptoms include flashbacks, nightmares, severe anxiety, and uncontrollable thoughts about the event. PTSD can affect individuals' daily functioning and is treated through therapy, medication, and support systems.

Predictive Analytics: Using statistical techniques and machine learning algorithms to analyze historical and current data to predict future outcomes and trends. Predictive analytics is used to forecast disease outbreaks, identify at-risk patients, optimize resource allocation, and improve patient outcomes through proactive interventions.

Primary Care Physician (PCP): A healthcare professional who is the first point of contact for patients seeking medical care. PCPs provide comprehensive and ongoing care, including preventive services, diagnosis and treatment of common conditions, and referrals to specialists when needed. They play a critical role in coordinating care and managing overall patient health.

Privacy Budget: A limit on the amount of information that can be revealed about input data when a computation is performed. It protects privacy and ensures the total amount of information disclosed stays within the defined bounds. It is crucial for protecting patient data in healthcare AI.

Problem-Oriented Medical Record (POMR): A structured approach to organizing medical information around a patient's health problems. It includes a problem list, patient data, and progress notes, often formatted using the SOAP method, enhancing clarity and communication in care.

Protected Health Information (PHI): Any health information that can be linked to a specific individual and is collected, stored, or transmitted by healthcare providers, health plans, and other covered entities. PHI includes medical records, billing information, and other identifiable health data and is protected under HIPAA to ensure privacy and security. PHI is a subset of Personal Identifiable Information.

Random Forests: An ensemble learning technique that builds multiple decision trees during training and aggregates their predictions for improved accuracy. Random Forests are widely used in healthcare for disease prediction and patient stratification tasks.

Real-World Data (RWD): Data related to patient health status and healthcare delivery collected from various sources outside clinical trials, including electronic health records, claims databases, patient registries, and wearable devices. RWD generates insights into treatment effectiveness, patient outcomes, and healthcare practices in real-world settings.

Real-World Evidence (RWE): Clinical evidence derived from real-world data analysis to evaluate the safety and efficacy of medical products, treatments, and interventions. RWE complements clinical trial data by providing insights into how treatments perform in broader, more diverse patient populations and real-world clinical settings.

Red Blood Cell (RBC): A type of blood cell that carries oxygen from the lungs to the rest of the body and returns carbon dioxide from the tissues to the lungs. RBCs contain hemoglobin, a protein that binds to oxygen, facilitating oxygen transport throughout the body. The number and function of RBCs are critical for assessing overall health and diagnosing conditions like anemia.

Reinforcement Learning from Human Feedback (RLHF): A machine learning (ML) technique that uses human feedback to optimize ML models to self-learn more efficiently. RLHF incorporates human feedback so the ML model can perform tasks more aligned with human goals, wants, and needs. RLHF is used throughout generative artificial intelligence applications, including in large language models.

Role-Based Access Control (RBAC): A security model that restricts system access based on the roles assigned to individuals within an organization. RBAC ensures that users have appropriate permissions, enhancing data security and minimizing the risk of unauthorized access to sensitive information. RBAC is commonly used to control electronic health record access.

Saliency Map: A visualization technique in computer vision that highlights important areas in an image for analysis by machine learning models. Saliency maps help identify critical regions in medical imaging, such as tumors or lesions.

Self-supervised Learning: A machine learning technique where models learn patterns from unlabeled data by solving pre-defined tasks. This approach is valuable in healthcare AI for processing large datasets, such as medical images and electronic health records, without requiring extensive manual labeling.

Shapley Additive exPlanations (SHAP): A method used to explain the output of machine learning models by attributing each feature's contribution to the prediction. SHAP values quantify the impact of individual features on the model's outcome, providing interpretability and transparency for complex models, which is essential for decision-making in healthcare.

Small-angle X-ray Scattering (SAXS): A technique used to study the structure of biological macromolecules, nanoparticles, and polymers in solution. SAXS measures the scattering of X-rays at small angles to provide information about the shape, size, and structural changes of molecules, making it a valuable tool in structural biology and materials science.

SOC 2 Type 2 Report: A report evaluating a company's internal controls for security, availability, processing integrity, confidentiality, and privacy. It is crucial for cloud service providers to ensure they protect customer data and meet compliance standards.

Social Determinants of Health (SDOH): Non-medical factors influencing health outcomes, including economic stability, education, social and community context, healthcare access, and neighborhood environment. SDOH impacts health disparities and are increasingly considered in healthcare delivery and policy to improve population health and reduce inequities.

Software as a Medical Device (SaMD): A software category that performs medical functions without being part of a physical medical device. SaMD is used for diagnosing, treating, or preventing disease and is regulated by government agencies to ensure safety and effectiveness. Examples include mobile applications that monitor vital signs or software that provides clinical decision support.

Subjective, Objective, Assessment, and Plan (SOAP): A standardized format for clinical documentation that organizes patient encounters into four parts: subjective (patient-reported concerns), objective (clinically observed data), assessment (diagnosis or impression), and plan (proposed treatments).

Supervised Learning: A machine learning technique where a model is trained on labeled datasets consisting of input-output pairs. The model learns to map the inputs to the correct outputs, enabling it to predict outcomes for new, unseen data. Supervised learning is widely used for diagnosing diseases, predicting patient outcomes, and detecting anomalies.

Surgical Site Infection (SSI): An infection that occurs at the site of a surgical incision within 30 days after surgery (or within a year if an implant is placed). SSIs are a common healthcare-associated infection and can lead to complications such as delayed wound healing, increased length of hospital stay, and higher healthcare costs. Prevention strategies include proper surgical techniques and infection control measures.

Synthetic Data: Artificially generated data that mimics real-world data, often created using AI techniques. Synthetic data is used to expand datasets for training machine learning models while protecting privacy and addressing data scarcity.

Targeted Real-time Early Warning System (TREWS): A predictive analytics system used in healthcare to provide early warnings for clinical deterioration or adverse events. TREWS combines patient data with advanced algorithms to identify patterns indicative of impending issues, allowing healthcare providers to intervene proactively and improve patient outcomes.

U.S. Department of Health and Human Services (HHS): The U.S. government agency responsible for protecting the health of all Americans and providing essential human services. HHS oversees various healthcare programs, including Medicare, Medicaid, and public health initiatives, and enforces regulations like HIPAA to ensure patient privacy and healthcare quality.

United States Medical Licensing Examination (USMLE): A three-step examination required for medical licensure in the United States. The USMLE assesses a physician's ability to apply medical knowledge, concepts, and principles to patient care and is a critical component in the licensing process for medical graduates.

Variational Autoencoder (VAE): A deep learning model for unsupervised learning tasks such as data generation and dimensionality reduction. VAEs consist of an encoder that compresses input data into a lower-dimensional space and a decoder that reconstructs the data, enabling the generation of new, similar data samples.

Virtual Assistant: An AI-powered software application designed to assist users by performing tasks, providing information, and facilitating communication. Virtual assistants can support clinicians and patients by scheduling appointments, managing clinical documentation, and providing health information.

Endnotes

https://barrychaiken.com/fh2050/endnotes

Chapter 2

Chaiken, B. P. (2024, September 6). Charting an ethical AI course: The LLM challenge in healthcare, Part 2. https://barrychaiken.com/archives/barrypchaiken/2024/09/529

Demner-Fushman, D., Kohli, M. D., Rosenman, M. B., Shooshan, S. E., Rodriguez, L., Antani, S., Thoma, G. R., & McDonald, C. J. (2016). Preparing a collection of radiology examinations for distribution and retrieval. *Journal of the American Medical Informatics Association*, 23(2), 304–310. https://doi.org/10.1093/jamia/ocv080

LeCun, Y., Bengio, Y., & Hinton, G. (2015). Deep learning. *Nature*, 521(7553), 436–444. https://doi.org/10.1038/nature14539

Ong, J. C. L., Chang, S. Y., William, W., Butte, A. J., Shah, N. H., Chew, L. S. T., Liu, N., Doshi-Velez, F., Lu, W., Savulescu, J., & Ting, D. S. W. (2024). Medical ethics of large language models in medicine. *NEJM AI*, 1(7). https://doi.org/10.1056/AIra2400038

Rajkomar, A., Dean, J., & Kohane, I. (2019). Machine learning in medicine. *The New England Journal of Medicine*, 380(14), 1347–1358. https://doi.org/10.1056/NEJMra1814259

Topol, E. J. (2019). High-performance medicine: The convergence of human and artificial intelligence. *Nature Medicine*, 25(1), 44–56. https://doi.org/10.1038/s41591-018-0300-7

Zech, J. R., Badgeley, M. A., Liu, M., Costa, A. B., Titano, J. J., & Oermann, E. K. (2018). Variable generalization performance of a deep learning model to detect pneumonia in chest radiographs: A cross-sectional study. *PLoS Medicine*, 15(11), e1002683. https://doi.org/10.1371/journal.pmed.1002683

Chapter 3

Aggarwal, R., Sounderajah, V., Martin, G., Ting, D. S. W., Karthikesalingam, A., King, D., ... Darzi, A. (2021). Diagnostic accuracy of deep learning in medical imaging: A systematic review and meta-analysis. *npj Digital Medicine*, 4(1), Article 23. https://doi.org/10.1038/s41746-021-00438-z

Beam, A. L., & Kohane, I. S. (2018). Big data and machine learning in health care. *JAMA*, 319(13), 1317–1318. https://doi.org/10.1001/jama.2017.18391

Chaiken, B. P. (2023, July 19). How computer vision and analytics is transforming medical imaging. https://barrychaiken.com/archives/barrypchaiken/2023/07/617

Esteva, A., Kuprel, B., Novoa, R. A., Ko, J., Swetter, S. M., Blau, H. M., & Thrun, S. (2017). Dermatologist-level classification of skin cancer with deep neural networks. *Nature*, 542(7639), 115–118. https://doi.org/10.1038/nature21056

He, J., Baxter, S. L., Xu, J., Xu, J., Zhou, X., & Zhang, K. (2019). The practical implementation of artificial intelligence technologies in medicine. *Nature Medicine*, 25(1), 30–36. https://doi.org/10.1038/s41591-018-0307-0

Litjens, G., Kooi, T., Bejnordi, B. E., Setio, A. A. A., Ciompi, F., Ghafoorian, M., ... Sánchez, C. I. (2017). A survey on deep learning in medical image analysis. *Medical Image Analysis*, 42, 60–88. https://doi.org/10.1016/j.media.2017.07.005

Rajkomar, A., Dean, J., & Kohane, I. (2019). Machine learning in medicine. *The New England Journal of Medicine*, 380(14), 1347–1358. https://doi.org/10.1056/NEJMra1814259

Topol, E. J. (2019). High-performance medicine: The convergence of human and artificial intelligence. *Nature Medicine*, 25(1), 44–56. https://doi.org/10.1038/s41591-018-0300-7

Xiao, C., Choi, E., & Sun, J. (2018). Opportunities and challenges in developing deep learning models using electronic health records data: A systematic review. *Journal of the American Medical Informatics Association*, 25(10), 1419–1428. https://doi.org/10.1093/jamia/ocy068

Yala, A., Lehman, C., Schuster, T., Portnoi, T., & Barzilay, R. (2019). A deep learning mammography-based model for improved breast cancer risk prediction. *Radiology*, 292(1), 60–66. https://doi.org/10.1148/radiol.2019182716

Chapter 4

Centers for Disease Control and Prevention. (2024, August 13). Hospital sepsis program core elements. *CDC*. https://www.cdc.gov/sepsis/hcp/core-elements/

Chaiken, B. P. (2023, August 28). Achieve value optimization by effectively leveraging analytics. https://barrychaiken.com/archives/barrypchaiken/2023/08/676

Char, D. S., Shah, N. H., & Magnus, D. (2018). Implementing machine learning in health care — Addressing ethical challenges. T*he New England Journal of Medicine*, 378(11), 981–983. https://doi.org/10.1056/NEJMp1714229

Gartner. (2016, June 12). The 360-degree approach to IT cost and value optimization. https://www.gartner.com/smarterwithgartner/the-360-degree-approach-to-it-cost-and-value-optimization

Massachusetts General Hospital. (n.d.). Patient safety and sepsis care. Retrieved November 24, 2024, from https://www.massgeneral.org/quality-and-safety/patient-safety/sepsis

Tjoa, E., & Guan, C. (2021). A survey on explainable artificial intelligence (XAI): Toward medical XAI. *IEEE Transactions on Neural Networks and Learning Systems*, 32(11), 4793–4813. https://doi.org/10.1109/TNNLS.2020.3027314

Chapter 5

Adams, R., Henry, K. E., Sridharan, A., Soleimani, H., Zhan, A., Rawat, N., Johnson, L., Hager, D. N., Cosgrove, S. E., Markowski, A., Klein, E. Y., Chen, E. S., Saheed, M. O., Henley, M., Miranda, S., Houston, K., Linton, R. C., Ahluwalia, A. R., Wu, A. W., & Saria, S. (2022). Prospective, multi-site study of patient outcomes after implementation of the TREWS machine learning-based early warning system for sepsis. *Nature Medicine*, 28(8), 1455–1460. https://doi.org/10.1038/s41591-022-01894-0

Baribeau, Y., Sharkey, A., Chaudhary, O., Krumm, S., Fatima, H., Mahmood, F., & Matyal, R. (2020). Handheld point-of-care ultrasound probes: The new generation of POCUS. *Journal of Cardiothoracic and Vascular Anesthesia,* 34(11), 3139–3145. https://doi.org/10.1053/j.jvca.2020.07.004

Chaiken, B. P. (2014, July 20). Railroads, weed and EHRs. https://barrychaiken.com/archives/barrypchaiken/2014/07/664

Haug, C. J., & Drazen, J. M. (2023). Artificial intelligence and machine learning in clinical medicine, 2023. *The New England Journal of Medicine*, 388(13), 1201–1208. https://doi.org/10.1056/NEJMra2302038

Hughes, M. S., Addala, A., & Buckingham, B. (2023). Digital technology for diabetes. *The New England Journal of Medicine*, 389(21), 2076–2086. https://doi.org/10.1056/NEJMra2215899

Jacobs, L. (2009). Interview with Lawrence Weed, MD—The father of the problem-oriented medical record looks ahead. *The Permanente Journal*, 13(3), 84–89. https://doi.org/10.7812/tpp/09-068

Rajpurkar, P., & Lungren, M. P. (2023). The current and future state of AI interpretation of medical images. *The New England Journal of Medicine*, 388(21), 1981–1990. https://doi.org/10.1056/NEJMra2301725

Sahni, N. R., & Carrus, B. (2023). Artificial intelligence in U.S. health care delivery. *The New England Journal of Medicine*, 389(4), 348–358. https://doi.org/10.1056/NEJMra2204673

Weed, L. L. (1964). Medical records, patient care, and medical education. *Irish Journal of Medical Science*, 39, 271–282. https://doi.org/10.1007/BF02945791

Weed, L. L. (1968). Medical records that guide and teach. *The New England Journal of Medicine*, 278(11), 593–600. https://doi.org/10.1056/NEJM196803142781105

Chapter 6

Chaiken, B. P. (2024, April 2). Transformative digital health tech: Focus on outcomes, privacy, workflow, data ownership. https://barrychaiken.com/archives/barrypchaiken/2024/04/356

Elkin, P. L., Mullin, S., Mardekian, J., Crowner, C., Sakilay, S., Sinha, S., Brady, G., Wright, M., Nolen, K., Trainer, J., Koppel, R., Schlegel, D., Kaushik, S., Zhao, J., Song, B., & Anand, E. (2021). Using artificial intelligence with natural language processing to combine electronic health record's structured and free text data to identify nonvalvular atrial fibrillation to decrease strokes and death: Evaluation and case-control study. *JMIR Medical Informatics*, 9(11), e28946. https://doi.org/10.2196/28946

Ginsburg, G. S., Picard, R. W., & Friend, S. H. (2024). Key issues as wearable digital health technologies enter clinical care. *The New England Journal of Medicine*, 390, 1118–1127. https://doi.org/10.1056/NEJMra2307160

Harris, J. E. (2023). An AI-enhanced electronic health record could boost primary care productivity. *JAMA*, 330(9), 801–802. https://doi.org/10.1001/jama.2023.14525

Hou, C., Carter, B., Hewitt, J., Francis, T., & Mayor, S. (2016). Do mobile phone applications improve glycemic control (HbA1c) in the self-management of diabetes? A systematic review, meta-analysis, and GRADE of 14 randomized trials. *Diabetes Care*, 39(11), 2089–2095. https://doi.org/10.2337/dc16-0346

Chapter 7

Chaiken, B. P. (2023, December 4). Understanding OpenAI's Q*: Are computers capable of thought experiments? https://barrychaiken.com/archives/barrypchaiken/2023/12/522

Char, D. S., Shah, N. H., & Magnus, D. (2018). Implementing machine learning in health care—Addressing ethical challenges. *The New England Journal of Medicine*, 378(11), 981–983. https://doi.org/10.1056/NEJMp1714229

Davenport, T., & Kalakota, R. (2019). The potential for artificial intelligence in healthcare. *Future Healthcare Journal*, 6(2), 94–98. https://doi.org/10.7861/futurehosp.6-2-94

Lee, P., Bubeck, S., & Petro, J. (2023). Benefits, limits, and risks of GPT-4 as an AI chatbot for medicine. *The New England Journal of Medicine*, 388, 1233–1239. https://doi.org/10.1056/NEJMsr2214184

Palmer, S. (2023, December 3). Understanding OpenAI's rumored humanity-ending algorithm. https://shellypalmer.com/2023/12/understanding-openais-rumored-humanity-ending-algorithm/

Rajkomar, A., Dean, J., & Kohane, I. (2019). Machine learning in medicine. *The New England Journal of Medicine*, 380, 1347–1358. https://doi.org/10.1056/NEJMra1814259

Reddy, S., Fox, J., & Purohit, M. P. (2019). Artificial intelligence-enabled healthcare delivery. *Journal of the Royal Society of Medicine*, 112(1), 22–28. https://doi.org/10.1177/0141076818815510

Topol, E. J. (2019). High-performance medicine: The convergence of human and artificial intelligence. *Nature Medicine*, 25, 44–56. https://doi.org/10.1038/s41591-018-0300-7

Vayena, E., Blasimme, A., & Cohen, I. G. (2018). Machine learning in medicine: Addressing ethical challenges. *PLOS Medicine*, 15(11), e1002689. https://doi.org/10.1371/journal.pmed.1002689

Chapter 8

Castro, M. A. A., de Santiago, I., Campbell, T. M., Vaughn, C., Hickey, T. E., Ross, E., Tilley, W. D., Markowetz, F., Ponder, B. A. J., & Meyer, K. B. (2016). Regulators of genetic risk of breast cancer identified by integrative network analysis. *Nature Genetics*, 48(1), 12–21. https://doi.org/10.1038/ng.3458

Chaiken, B. P. (2024, May 12). Collaborative intelligence: How human expertise and AI synergize in healthcare. https://barrychaiken.com/archives/barrypchaiken/2024/05/351

Ching, T., Himmelstein, D. S., Beaulieu-Jones, B. K., Kalinin, A. A., Do, B. T., Way, G. P., Ferrero, E., Agapow, P.-M., Zietz, M., Hoffman, M. M., Xie, W., Rosen, G. L., Lengerich, B. J., Israeli, J., Lanchantin, J., Woloszynek, S., Carpenter, A. E., Shrikumar, A., Xu, J., ... Greene, C. S. (2018). Opportunities and obstacles for deep learning in biology and medicine. *Journal of the Royal Society Interface*, 15(141), Article 20170387. https://doi.org/10.1098/rsif.2017.0387

De Leo, A., Bloxsome, D., & Bayes, S. (2023). Approaches to clinical guideline development in healthcare: A scoping review and document analysis. *BMC Health Services Research*, 23, 37. https://doi.org/10.1186/s12913-022-08975-3

Fogel, D. B. (2018). Factors associated with clinical trials that fail and opportunities for improving the likelihood of success: A review. Contemporary *Clinical Trials Communications*, 11, 156–164. https://doi.org/10.1016/j.conctc.2018.08.001

Google. (2024, May 8). Google DeepMind and Isomorphic Labs introduce AlphaFold 3 AI model. *The Keyword*. https://blog.google/technology/ai/google-deepmind-isomorphic-alphafold-3-ai-model/

Google DeepMind. (n.d.). AlphaFold. *Google DeepMind*. Retrieved November 24, 2024, from https://deepmind.google/technologies/alphafold/

Harrer, S., Shah, P., Antony, B., & Hu, J. (2019). Artificial intelligence for clinical trial design. *Trends in Pharmacological Sciences*, 40(8), 577–591. https://doi.org/10.1016/j.tips.2019.05.005

Hernandez, A. F., & Lindsell, C. J. (2023). The future of clinical trials: Artificial to augmented to applied intelligence. *JAMA*, 330(21), 2061–2063. https://doi.org/10.1001/jama.2023.23822

Hunter, D. J., & Holmes, C. (2023). Where medical statistics meets artificial intelligence. *The New England Journal of Medicine*, 389, 1211–1219. https://doi.org/10.1056/NEJMra2212850

Jumper, J., & Hassabis, D. (2023). The protein structure prediction revolution and its implications for medicine: 2023 Albert Lasker Basic Medical Research Award. *JAMA*, 330(15), 1425–1426. https://doi.org/10.1001/jama.2023.17095

Jumper, J., Evans, R., Pritzel, A., Green, T., Figurnov, M., Ronneberger, O., Tunyasuvunakool, K., Bates, R., Žídek, A., Potapenko, A., Bridgland, A., Meyer, C., Kohl, S. A. A., Ballard, A. J., Cowie, A., Romera-Paredes, B., Nikolov, S.,

Jain, R., Adler, J., ... Hassabis, D. (2021). Highly accurate protein structure prediction with AlphaFold. *Nature*, 596(7873), 583–589. https://doi.org/10.1038/s41586-021-03819-2

Mak, K.-K., & Pichika, M. R. (2019). Artificial intelligence in drug development: Present status and future prospects. *Drug Discovery Today*, 24(3), 773–780. https://doi.org/10.1016/j.drudis.2018.11.014

Mosalaganti, S., Obarska-Kosinska, A., Siggel, M., Turonova, B., Zimmerli, C. E., Buczak, K., Schmidt, F. H., Margiotta, E., Mackmull, M.-T., Hagen, W., Hummer, G., Beck, M., & Kosinski, J. (2021). Artificial intelligence reveals nuclear pore complexity. *bioRxiv*. https://doi.org/10.1101/2021.10.26.465776

Obermeyer, Z., Powers, B., Vogeli, C., & Mullainathan, S. (2019). Dissecting racial bias in an algorithm used to manage the health of populations. *Science*, 366(6464), 447–453. https://doi.org/10.1126/science.aax2342

Palmer, S. (2024, May 5). Who is really training your AI? The role of SMEs in AI data annotation. https://shellypalmer.com/2024/05/who-is-really-training-your-ai-the-role-of-smes-in-ai-data-annotation/

Senior, A. W., Evans, R., Jumper, J., Kirkpatrick, J., Sifre, L., Green, T., Qin, C., Žídek, A., Nelson, A. W. R., Bridgland, A., Penedones, H., Petersen, S., Simonyan, K., Crossan, S., Jones, D. T., Silver, D., Kavukcuoglu, K., Hassabis, D., & Kohli, P. (2020). Improved protein structure prediction using potentials from deep learning. *Nature*, 577(7792), 706–710. https://doi.org/10.1038/s41586-019-1923-7

Smalley, E. (2017). AI-powered drug discovery captures pharma interest. *Nature Biotechnology*, 35(7), 604–605. https://doi.org/10.1038/nbt0717-604

Suran, M., & Hswen, Y. (2024). How do policymakers regulate AI and accommodate innovation in research and medicine? *JAMA*, 331(3), 185–187. https://doi.org/10.1001/jama.2023.22625

Tschandl, P., Rinner, C., Apalla, Z., Argenziano, G., Codella, N., Halpern, A., Kittler, H., Lallas, A., Longo, C., Malvehy, J., Puig, S., Rosendahl, C., Soyer, H. P., & Zalaudek, I. (2020). Human–computer collaboration for skin cancer recognition. *Nature Medicine*, 26, 1229–1234. https://doi.org/10.1038/s41591-020-0942-0

Tunyasuvunakool, K., Adler, J., Wu, Z., Green, T., Zielinski, M., Žídek, A., Bridgland, A., Cowie, A., Meyer, C., Laydon, A., Velankar, S., Kleywegt, G. J., Bateman, A., Evans, R., Pritzel, A., Figurnov, M., Ronneberger, O., Kohl, S. A. A., Potapenko, A., ... Hassabis, D. (2021). Highly accurate protein structure prediction for the human proteome. *Nature*, 596(7873), 590–596. https://doi.org/10.1038/s41586-021-03828-1

Turing. (n.d.). Fine-tuning LLMs: Overview, methods, and best practices. *Turing*. Retrieved November 24, 2024, from https://www.turing.com/resources/finetuning-large-language-models

Vamathevan, J., Clark, D., Czodrowski, P., Dunham, I., Ferran, E., Lee, G., Li, B., Madabhushi, A., Shah, P., Spitzer, M., & Zhao, S. (2019). Applications of machine learning in drug discovery and development. *Nature Reviews Drug Discovery*, 18(6), 463–477. https://doi.org/10.1038/s41573-019-0024-5

Wacker, D., Stevens, R. C., & Roth, B. L. (2017). How ligands illuminate GPCR molecular pharmacology. *Cell*, 170(3), 414–427. https://doi.org/10.1016/j.cell.2017.07.009

Weissman, G. E., & Joynt Maddox, K. E. (2023). Guiding risk adjustment models toward machine learning methods. *JAMA*, 330(9), 807–808. https://doi.org/10.1001/jama.2023.12920

Chapter 9

Ayers, J. W., Desai, N., & Smith, D. M. (2024). Regulate artificial intelligence in health care by prioritizing patient outcomes. *JAMA*, 331(8), 639–640. https://doi.org/10.1001/jama.2024.0549

Blum, D. (2024, March 16). Health misinformation is evolving. Here's how to spot it. *The New York Times*. https://www.nytimes.com/2024/03/16/well/health-misinformation.html

Chaiken, B. P. (2024, March 20). Protect patients from AI-driven healthcare misinformation. https://barrychaiken.com/archives/barrypchaiken/2024/03/357

Goddard, K., Roudsari, A., & Wyatt, J. C. (2011). Automation bias: A systematic review of frequency, effect mediators, and mitigators. *Journal of the American Medical Informatics Association*, 19(1), 121–27. https://doi.org/10.1136/amiajnl-2011-000089

Johnson, A. E. W., Ghassemi, M. M., Nemati, S., Niehaus, K. E., Clifton, D. A., & Clifford, G. D. (2016). Machine learning and decision support in critical care. *Proceedings of the IEEE Institute of Electrical and Electronics Engineers*, 104(2), 444–466. https://doi.org/10.1109/JPROC.2015.2501978

Liptak, A. (2024, March 18). Supreme Court wary of states' bid to limit federal contact with social media companies. *The New York Times*. https://www.nytimes.com/2024/03/18/us/politics/supreme-court-white-house-misinformation.html

Nijman, J., Zoodsma, R. S., & Koomen, E. (2024). A strategy for artificial intelligence with clinical impact—Eyes on the prize. *JAMA Pediatrics*, 178(3), 219–220. https://doi.org/10.1001/jamapediatrics.2023.6259

Wilson, P., Crowe, B., Abdulnour, R.-E., & Rodman, A. (2024). Clinical reasoning of a generative artificial intelligence model compared with physicians. *JAMA Internal Medicine*, 184(5), 581–583. https://doi.org/10.1001/jamainternmed.2023.7962

Rajkomar, A., Oren, E., Chen, K., Dai, A. M., Hajaj, N., Hardt, M., Liu, P. J., Liu, X., Marcus, J., Sun, M., Sundberg, P., Yee, H., Zhang, K., Zhang, Y., Flores, G., Duggan, G. E., Irvine, J., Le, Q., Litsch, K., … Corrado, G. S. (2018). Scalable and accurate deep learning with electronic health records. *NPJ Digital Medicine*, 1, Article 18. https://doi.org/10.1038/s41746-018-0029-1

Safavi, K. C., Khaniyev, T., Copenhaver, M., Seelen, M., Zenteno Langle, A. C., Zanger, J., Daily, B., Levi, R., & Dunn, P. (2019). Development and validation of a machine learning model to aid discharge processes for inpatient surgical care. *JAMA Network Open*, 2(12), e1917221. https://doi.org/10.1001/jamanetworkopen.2019.17221

Sarkar, U., & Bates, D. W. (2024). Using artificial intelligence to improve primary care for patients and clinicians. *JAMA Internal Medicine*, 184(4), 343–344. https://doi.org/10.1001/jamainternmed.2023.7965

Topol, E. J. (2019). High-performance medicine: The convergence of human and artificial intelligence. *Nature Medicine*, 25, 44–56. https://doi.org/10.1038/s41591-018-0300-7

Vellido, A. (2020). The importance of interpretability and visualization in machine learning for applications in medicine and health care. *Neural Computing and Applications*, 32, 18069–18083. https://doi.org/10.1007/s00521-019-04051-w

Chapter 10

Abbasi, J., & Hswen, Y. (2024). Blind spots, shortcuts, and automation bias—Researchers are aiming to improve AI clinical models. *JAMA*, 331(11), 903–906. https://doi.org/10.1001/jama.2023.28262

Accenture. (2022). Artificial intelligence: Healthcare's new nervous system. https://www.accenture.com/us-en/insights/health/artificial-intelligence-healthcare

Berwick, D. M. (2023). Salve lucrum: The existential threat of greed in US health care. *JAMA*, 329(8), 629–630. https://doi.org/10.1001/jama.2023.0846

Chaiken, B. P. (2024, March 4). Navigating risk: Standards required for AI-generated clinical summaries. https://barrychaiken.com/archives/barrypchaiken/2024/03/360

Goodman, K. E., Yi, P. H., & Morgan, D. J. (2024). AI-generated clinical summaries require more than accuracy. *JAMA*, 331(8), 637–638. https://doi.org/10.1001/jama.2024.0555

Harris, J. E. (2023). AI-enhanced electronic health record could boost primary care productivity. *JAMA*, 330(9), 801–802. https://doi.org/10.1001/jama.2023.14525

Khera, R., Simon, M. A., & Ross, J. S. (2023). Automation bias and assistive AI: Risk of harm from AI-driven clinical decision support. *JAMA*, 330(23), 2255–2257. https://doi.org/10.1001/jama.2023.22557

Sarkar, U., & Bates, D. W. (2024). Using artificial intelligence to improve primary care for patients and clinicians. *JAMA Internal Medicine*, 184(4), 343–344. https://doi.org/10.1001/jamainternmed.2023.7965

U.S. Food and Drug Administration. (n.d.). Software as a medical device (SaMD). *FDA*. Retrieved November 24, 2024, from https://www.fda.gov/medical-devices/digital-health-center-excellence/software-medical-device-samd

Chapter 11

Chaiken, B. P. (2024, April 4). Why every healthcare organization needs a chief AI officer. https://barrychaiken.com/archives/barrypchaiken/2024/04/353

Davenport, T., & Kalakota, R. (2019). The potential for artificial intelligence in healthcare. *Future Healthcare Journal*, 6(2), 94–98. https://doi.org/10.7861/futurehosp.6-2-94

Fogo, A. B., Kronbichler, A., & Bajema, I. M. (2024). AI's threat to the medical profession. *JAMA*, 331(6), 471–472. https://doi.org/10.1001/jama.2024.0018

McKinney, S. M., Sieniek, M., Godbole, V., Godwin, J., Antropova, N., Ashrafian, H., Back, T., Chesus, M., Corrado, G. S., Darzi, A., Etemadi, M., Garcia-Vicente, F., Gilbert, F. J., Halling-Brown, M., Hassabis, D., Jansen, S., Karthikesalingam, A., Kelly, C. J., King, D., ... Shetty, S. (2020). International evaluation of an AI system for breast cancer screening. *Nature*, 577(7788), 89–94. https://doi.org/10.1038/s41586-019-1799-6

Chapter 12

BBC News. (2024). *Hackers expose deep cybersecurity vulner-abilities in AI* [Video]. YouTube. https://www.youtube.com/watch?v=Fg9hCKH1sYs

Chaiken, B. P. (2024, July 8). Will hackers derail AI-driven healthcare? https://barrychaiken.com/archives/barrypchaiken/2024/07/387

Department for Science, Innovation and Technology, & AI Safety Institute. (2024, May 17). International scientific report on the safety of advanced AI: An up-to-date, evidence-based report on the science of advanced artificial intelligence (AI) safety. *GOV.UK*. https://www.gov.uk/government/publications/international-scientific-report-on-the-safety-of-advanced-ai

Festival Of The Sun. (2024). *Jack Dorsey – Tech and freedom* [Video]. YouTube. https://www.youtube.com/watch?v=t-40158eRqo

Kanter, G. P., & Packel, E. A. (2023). Health care privacy risks of AI chatbots. *JAMA*, 330(4), 311–312. https://doi.org/10.1001/jama.2023.9618

Lee, P., Bubeck, S., & Petro, J. (2023). Benefits, limits, and risks of GPT-4 as an AI chatbot for medicine. *The New England Journal of Medicine*, 388(13), 1223–1239. https://doi.org/10.1056/NEJMsr2214184

Garfinkel, S., Guttman, B., Near, J., Dajani, A. N., & Singer, P. (2023). *De-identifying government datasets: Techniques and governance (NIST Special Publication 800-188)*. National Institute of Standards and Technology. https://doi.org/10.6028/NIST.SP.800-188

Reed, J. (2024, May 8). Change Healthcare attack expected to exceed $1 billion in costs. *Security Intelligence*. https://securityintelligence.com/news/change-healthcare-cyberattack-exceeds-1-billion-costs

U.S. Department of Health and Human Services. (n.d.). Breach notification rule. *HHS.gov*. Retrieved November 24, 2024, from https://www.hhs.gov/hipaa/for-professionals/breach-notification/index.html

Chapter 13

Ayers, J. W., Desai, N., & Smith, D. M. (2024). Regulate artificial intelligence in health care by prioritizing patient outcomes. *JAMA*, 331(8), 639–640. https://doi.org/10.1001/jama.2023.27449

Blum, D. (2024, March 16). Health misinformation is evolving. Here's how to spot it. *The New York Times*. https://www.nytimes.com/2024/03/16/well/health-misinformation.html

Chaiken, B. P. (2024, February 22). Legal liability of healthcare AI: How do we protect patients? https://barrychaiken.com/archives/barrypchaiken/2024/02/362

Challen, R., Denny, J., Pitt, M., Gompels, L., Edwards, T., & Tsaneva-Atanasova, K. (2019). Artificial intelligence, bias and clinical safety. *BMJ Quality & Safety*, 28(3), 231–237. https://doi.org/10.1136/bmjqs-2018-008370

Ghassemi, M., Oakden-Rayner, L., & Beam, A. L. (2021). The false hope of current approaches to explainable artificial intelligence in health care. *The Lancet Digital Health*, 3(11), e745–e750. https://doi.org/10.1016/S2589-7500(21)00208-9

Goodman, K. E., Yi, P. H., & Morgan, D. J. (2024). AI-generated clinical summaries require more than accuracy. *JAMA*, 331(8), 637–638. https://doi.org/10.1001/jama.2023.27450

He, J., Baxter, S. L., Xu, J., Xu, J., Zhou, X., & Zhang, K. (2019). The practical implementation of artificial intelligence technologies in medicine. *Nature Medicine*, 25(1), 30–36. https://doi.org/10.1038/s41591-018-0307-0

IBM. (n.d.). What is explainable AI? *IBM*. Retrieved November 24, 2024, from https://www.ibm.com/topics/explainable-ai

Jabbour, S., Fouhey, D., Shepard, S., Syed, Z., Malani, P. N., Wiens, J., & Nallamothu, B. K. (2023). Measuring the impact of AI in the diagnosis of hospitalized patients: A randomized clinical vignette survey study. *JAMA*, 330(23), 2285–2293. https://doi.org/10.1001/jama.2023.23604

Kelly, C. J., Karthikesalingam, A., Suleyman, M., et al. (2019). Key challenges for delivering clinical impact with artificial intelligence. *BMC Medicine*, 17(1), Article 195. https://doi.org/10.1186/s12916-019-1426-2

Khera, R., Simon, M. A., & Ross, J. S. (2023). Automation bias and assistive AI: Risk of harm from AI-driven clinical decision support. *JAMA*, 330(23), 2255–2257. https://doi.org/10.1001/jama.2023.23654

Lee, P., Bubeck, S., & Petro, J. (2023). Benefits, limits, and risks of GPT-4 as an AI chatbot for medicine. *The New England Journal of Medicine*, 388(13), 1223–1239. https://doi.org/10.1056/NEJMsr2214184

Mello, M. M., & Guha, N. (2024). Understanding liability risk from using health care artificial intelligence tools. *The New England Journal of Medicine*, 390(3), 271–278. https://doi.org/10.1056/NEJMhle2308901

Topol, E. J. (2019). High-performance medicine: The convergence of human and artificial intelligence. *Nature Medicine*, 25(1), 44–56. https://doi.org/10.1038/s41591-018-0300-7

Chapter 14

American Medical Association. (2023, November 28). AMA issues new principles for AI development, deployment & use. *AMA*. https://www.ama-assn.org/press-center/press-releases/ama-issues-new-principles-ai-development-deployment-use

Chaiken, B. P. (2024, April 29). The price of progress: Protecting patient privacy in the age of AI. https://barrychaiken.com/archives/barrypchaiken/2024/04/352

Dorr, D. A., Adams, L., & Embí, P. J. (2023). Harnessing the promise of artificial intelligence responsibly. *JAMA*, 329(16), 1347–1348. https://doi.org/10.1001/jama.2023.2771

Ferryman, K., Mackintosh, M., & Ghassemi, M. (2023). Considering biased data as informative artifacts in AI-assisted health care. *The New England Journal of Medicine*, 389(9), 833–838. https://doi.org/10.1056/NEJMra2214964

Mello, M. M., & Guha, N. (2023). Biden's executive order on AI: Implications for health care. *JAMA*, 330(23), 2281–2283. https://doi.org/10.1001/jama.2023.23605

Metz, C., Kang, C., Frenkel, S., Thompson, S. A., & Grant, N. (2024, April 6). How tech giants cut corners to harvest data for A.I. *The New York Times*. https://www.nytimes.com/2024/04/06/technology/tech-giants-harvest-data-artificial-intelligence.html

Neumann, P. J., & Tunis, S. R. (2023). Turning CMS into a health technology assessment organization. *The New England Journal of Medicine*, 389(8), 682–684. https://doi.org/10.1056/NEJMp2305280

The White House. (2022). *Blueprint for an AI Bill of Rights: Making automated systems work for the American people.* https://www.whitehouse.gov/ostp/ai-bill-of-rights/

U.S. Food and Drug Administration. (n.d.). Software as a medical device (SaMD). *FDA*. Retrieved November 24, 2024, from

https://www.fda.gov/medical-devices/
digital-health-center-excellence/software-medical-device-samd

Chapter 15

Chaiken, B. P. (2024, July 19). Beyond black box healthcare AI: Gain trust with transparency. https://barrychaiken.com/archives/barrypchaiken/2024/07/125

European Commission. (2017). *Attitudes towards the impact of digitisation and automation on daily life: Report. Publications Office of the European Union.* https://data.europa.eu/doi/10.2759/835661

Biden, J. R. (2023). *Executive Order 14110: Safe, secure, and trustworthy development and use of artificial intelligence. Federal Register.* https://www.federalregister.gov/documents/2023/11/01/2023-24283/safe-secure-and-trustworthy-development-and-use-of-artificial-intelligence

Ferryman, K., Mackintosh, M., & Ghassemi, M. (2023). Considering biased data as informative artifacts in AI-assisted health care. *The New England Journal of Medicine, 389,* 833–838. https://doi.org/10.1056/NEJMra2214964

Hotez, P. J. (2024). Health disinformation—Gaining strength, becoming infinite. *JAMA Internal Medicine, 184*(1), 96–97. https://doi.org/10.1001/jamainternmed.2023.5946

Mello, M. M., Shah, N. H., & Char, D. S. (2024). President Biden's executive order on artificial intelligence—Implications for health care organizations. *JAMA, 331*(1), 17–18. https://doi.org/10.1001/jama.2023.25051

Menz, B. D., Modi, N. D., Sorich, M. J., & Hopkins, A. M. (2024). Health disinformation use case highlighting the urgent need for artificial intelligence vigilance: Weapons of mass disinformation. *JAMA Internal Medicine, 184*(1), 92–96. https://doi.org/10.1001/jamainternmed.2023.5947

Office of the National Coordinator for Health Information Technology. (2023, December). *Decision support interventions (DSI) fact sheet.* U.S. Department of Health and Human Services. https://www.healthit.gov/sites/default/files/page/2023-12/HTI-1_DSI_fact%20sheet_508.pdf

Shah, N. H., Halamka, J. D., Saria, S., Pencina, M., Tazbaz, T., Tripathi, M., Callahan, A., Hildahl, H., & Anderson, B. (2024). A nationwide network of health AI assurance laboratories. *JAMA, 331*(3), 245–249. https://doi.org/10.1001/jama.2023.26930

Sim, I., & Cassel, C. (2024). The ethics of relational AI — Expanding and implementing the Belmont principles. *The New England Journal of Medicine*, 391, 193–196. https://doi.org/10.1056/NEJMp231477

Zhang, B., & Dafoe, A. (2019). Artificial intelligence: American attitudes and trends. *SSRN*. https://doi.org/10.2139/ssrn.3312874

Chapter 16

Chaiken, B. P. (2023, June 5). Turn and face the strange, changes. https://barry-chaiken.com/archives/barrypchaiken/2023/06/643

Davenport, T., & Kalakota, R. (2019). The potential for artificial intelligence in healthcare. *Future Healthcare Journal*, 6(2), 94–98. https://doi.org/10.7861/futurehosp.6-2-94

Esteva, A., Kuprel, B., Novoa, R., Ko, J., Swetter, S. M., Blau, H. M., & Thrun, S. (2017). Dermatologist-level classification of skin cancer with deep neural networks. *Nature*, 542(7639), 115–118. https://doi.org/10.1038/nature21056

He, J., Baxter, S. L., Xu, J., Xu, J., & Zhou, X. (2019). The practical implementation of artificial intelligence technologies in medicine. *Nature Medicine*, 25, 30–36. https://doi.org/10.1038/s41591-018-0307-0

Liu, X., Faes, L., Kale, A. U., Wagner, S. K., Fu, D. J., Bruynseels, A., Mahendiran, T., Moraes, G., Shamdas, M., Kern, C., Ledsam, J. R., Schmid, M. K., Balaskas, K., Topol, E. J., Bachmann, L. M., Keane, P. A., & Denniston, A. K. (2019). A comparison of deep learning performance against health-care professionals in detecting diseases from medical imaging: A systematic review and meta-analysis. *The Lancet Digital Health*, 1(6), e271–e297. https://doi.org/10.1016/S2589-7500(19)30123-2

Rajkomar, A., Dean, J., & Kohane, I. (2019). Machine learning in medicine. *The New England Journal of Medicine*, 380(14), 1347–1358. https://doi.org/10.1056/NEJMra1814259

Shortliffe, E. H., & Sepúlveda, M. J. (2018). Clinical decision support in the era of artificial intelligence. *JAMA*, 320(21), 2199–2200. https://doi.org/10.1001/jama.2018.17163

Topol, E. J. (2019). High-performance medicine: The convergence of human and artificial intelligence. *Nature Medicine*, 25(1), 44–56. https://doi.org/10.1038/s41591-018-0300-7

Wiens, J., Saria, S., Sendak, M., Ghassemi, M., Liu, V. X., Doshi-Velez, F., Jung, K., Heller, K., Kale, D., Saeed, M., Ossorio, P. N., Thadaney-Israni, S., & Goldenberg, A. (2019). Do no harm: A roadmap for responsible machine learning for health care. *Nature Medicine*, 25, 1337–1340. https://doi.org/10.1038/s41591-019-0548-6

Yu, K. H., Beam, A. L., & Kohane, I. S. (2018). Artificial intelligence in healthcare. *Nature Biomedical Engineering*, 2, 719–731. https://doi.org/10.1038/s41551-018-0305-z

Chapter 17

Ayers, J. W., Desai, N., & Smith, D. M. (2024). Regulate artificial intelligence in health care by prioritizing patient outcomes. *JAMA*, 331(8), 639–640. https://doi.org/10.1001/jama.2024.0549

Bates, D. W., Saria, S., Ohno-Machado, L., Shah, A., & Escobar, G. (2014). Big data in health care: Using analytics to identify and manage high-risk and high-cost patients. *Health Affairs*, 33(7), 1123–1131. https://doi.org/10.1377/hlthaff.2014.0041

Chaiken, B. P. (2024, March 11). Setting the standard: The critical role of outcome-centric healthcare AI regulation. https://barrychaiken.com/archives/barrypchaiken/2024/03/359

Davenport, T., & Kalakota, R. (2019). The potential for artificial intelligence in healthcare. *Future Healthcare Journal*, 6(2), 94–98. https://doi.org/10.7861/futurehosp.6-2-94

Lehman, W. E. K., Greener, J. M., & Simpson, D. D. (2002). Assessing organizational readiness for change. *Journal of Substance Abuse Treatment*, 22(4), 197–209. https://doi.org/10.1016/S0740-5472(02)00233-7

Weiner, B. J. (2009). A theory of organizational readiness for change. *Implementation Science*, 4, Article 67. https://doi.org/10.1186/1748-5908-4-67

Wong, A., Otles, E., Donnelly, J. P., Krumm, A., McCullough, J., DeTroyer-Cooley, O., Pestrue, J., Phillips, M., Konye, J., Penoza, C., Ghous, M., & Singh, K. (2021). External validation of a widely implemented proprietary sepsis prediction model in hospitalized patients. *JAMA Internal Medicine*, 181(8), 1065–1070. https://doi.org/10.1001/jamainternmed.2021.2626

Acknowledgments

Just a machine to make big decisions,
Programmed by fellows with compassion and vision.
We'll be clean when their work is done;
We'll be eternally free, yes, and eternally young.
What a beautiful world this will be,
What a glorious time to be free.

—From "I.G.Y. (International Geophysical Year)" by
Donald Fagen, 1982, The Nightfly. Warner Records.

These lyrics from Donald Fagen's vision of the future serve as
a perfect gateway into the story of this book. Just as the International Geophysical Year (IGY) represented a time of unprecedented
scientific collaboration and discovery, today's healthcare artificial
intelligence (AI) stands at a similar frontier. While Fagen's lyrics playfully captured the optimistic futurism of the 1950s, they
unknowingly predicted our present moment, where machines truly
are making big decisions—not with the naive optimism of past
decades, but through careful development by researchers, clinicians,
and technologists who bring both compassion and vision to their
work. This book emerged from my belief that properly developed
and thoughtfully deployed artificial intelligence will help create that
beautiful world in healthcare, not by replacing human judgment but
by enhancing our ability to care for one another.

The journey of writing this book parallels the evolution of AI
in healthcare itself—from a promising concept to a practical reality.

Like the scientists of the IGY who mapped our oceans and studied our atmosphere, today's healthcare AI pioneers are charting new territories in medical diagnosis, treatment planning, and patient care. But unlike the sometimes-unbridled optimism of the 1950s that Fagen gently satirized, our current moment demands a more nuanced vision. We learned that the *big decisions* these machines make must be guided by clinical expertise, ethical considerations, and, above all, a deep understanding of human needs. The fellows with *compassion and vision* in today's healthcare AI world are not just programmers and engineers but also doctors, nurses, medical researchers, ethicists, and patients—all contributing their insights to ensure that AI serves healthcare's fundamental mission: improving human lives.

No work of this magnitude is possible without unwavering personal support, and my deepest gratitude goes to my wife, Beka. Her patience, understanding, and encouragement sustained me through countless hours of writing, research, and revision. As a pediatric nurse who has dedicated her career to both intensive care and ambulatory pediatrics, Beka brings a profound understanding of healthcare's human dimension to everything she touches. She created the space I needed to complete this work and served as a vital sounding board, offering perspectives that helped ground this book in the reality of frontline healthcare rather than pure technology. Her belief in the importance of this project, even during its most challenging moments, made its completion possible. Through late nights and long weekends, her support never wavered, reminding me why making healthcare more effective through AI matters— because, at its heart, it is about supporting healthcare heroes like her who work tirelessly, caring for our most vulnerable patients and their families. I hope this book helps make their noble work just a little bit easier.

I am deeply grateful to Dr. David Gute, Professor of Public Health and Community Medicine at Tufts University, whose insights and friendship helped shape this work in uniquely mean-ingful ways. Our monthly *walkie-talkies* around Boston became an invaluable intellectual journey, where our wide-ranging conversa-tions evolved naturally with each step taken. These walking discus-sions provided not just exercise for the body but essential exercise for the mind, offering fresh perspectives and a deeper understanding of how AI can serve healthcare and education. His subsequent review of the manuscript brought the same thoughtful consideration that characterized our walks, helping to ensure the book's ideas were as clear and impactful as our conversations. David's ability to blend academic rigor with practical wisdom exemplifies the multidisci-plinary thinking that healthcare AI demands.

I owe a special debt of gratitude to Tom Koulopoulos, whose mentorship proved invaluable throughout this project. As a trusted advisor who encouraged me to build upon the foundation laid in my first book, *Navigating the Code*, Tom's experienced guidance helped shape not just the structure of this book but its very existence. Drawing from his experience as the author of more than a dozen books, his expert guidance on structure and content development proved invaluable, helping to shape this complex topic into a coher-ent and engaging narrative. His mentorship encourages profession-als to write books that share their unique expertise and perspectives and inspires them to step onto keynote stages, helping industry leaders transform their knowledge into powerful stories that drive positive change within their organizations.

I am indebted to a remarkable group of reviewers whose diverse expertise significantly enhanced this book's depth and reach. Dr. Joseph Restuccia, Professor of Operations & Technol-ogy Management at Boston University, contributed his profound understanding of healthcare business operations, helping ensure the book addressed the real-world complexities of implementing AI in healthcare settings. Dr. Roger Flint brought invaluable healthcare insights shaped by his experiences as a physician and entrepreneur in the United Kingdom, offering perspectives that helped bridge the gap between medical practice and innovation. Jeff Huckaby's deep expertise in analytics and entrepreneurial spirit provided crucial guidance in explaining complex technical concepts while always offering encouragement when needed. Ben Breeze, contributing from London, brought his healthcare consulting acumen to bear on the content and ensure the book's practical relevance and reach.

I am grateful to Cliff Matthews, whose monthly coffee conversations became cherished interludes of insight and reflection. With his deep expertise in coffee and wine, Cliff brought an appreciation for life's subtle complexities to our discussions, reminding me that the richest ideas, like the finest beverages, emerge from careful cultivation and mindful discourse.

Writing a book can be a solitary endeavor, which makes friendship all the more precious during the process. I want to thank Dr. Hal Wolfson, whose rediscovered friendship from our high school days brought not just fresh energy and perspective, but also warmth and camaraderie to this project. Sometimes, the best insights come from conversations with those who knew us before our professional journeys began.

A special note of appreciation goes to *LGM* and *OMG* for providing a welcome distraction and unexpected inspiration during the writing process. Their energy and spirit offered necessary mental breaks, allowing me to return to the manuscript with renewed focus and vigor. More than just entertainment, they demonstrated the principles that resonated deeply with my work: the power of believing in a process, maintaining a positive focus, and persevering until reaching the goal. These letters carry special meaning for those who know—a shared language of persistence, hope, and unwavering belief in what is possible when you never give up on the vision.

I would be mindful to acknowledge the AI tools that assisted in the technical aspects of creating this book. *Claude* and *ChatGPT* served as valuable research assistants, helping to verify information and offering different perspectives on complex topics. *Grammarly's* assistance with editing and clarity helped refine the manuscript's language. While these tools provided technical support, all ideas, analyses, and conclusions in this book remain my own. The use of these AI assistants in writing a book about AI in healthcare seems particularly fitting—demonstrating both the practical benefits and limitations of artificial intelligence as a complement to human creativity and expertise.

As I close these acknowledgments, I am struck by how this book's journey reflects the very essence of technological progress—a tapestry woven from individual contributions, collaborative insights, and shared aspirations for a better future. Just as artificial intelligence in healthcare works best when it enhances and supports human capability, this book emerged from an incredible synergy of human connections, expertise, and encouragement. To everyone who contributed to this journey, whether named in these pages or touching the project in ways large and small, thank you for helping to illuminate the path toward a healthcare future that is both more capable and more compassionate.

–30–

Barry P. Chaiken, MD
Boston, MA
December 5, 2024

About the Author

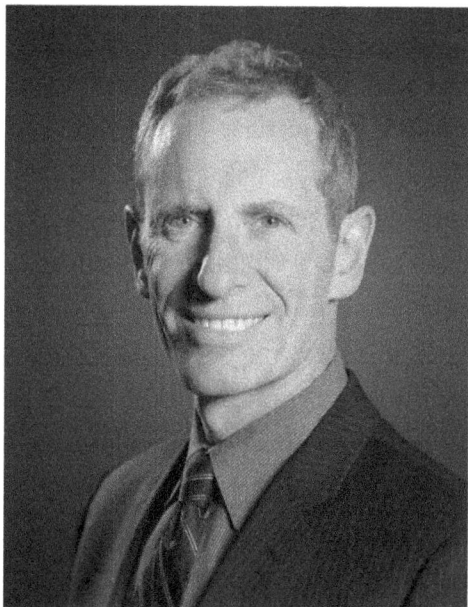

Barry P. Chaiken, MD, MPH, is a distinguished figure at the intersection of healthcare innovation and technology, with over 25 years dedicated to advancing healthcare information technology, clinical transformation, and the strategic use of data to enhance patient safety and healthcare outcomes. As a pioneering physician innovator and a leading expert in artificial intelligence in healthcare, Dr. Chaiken's contributions have significantly influenced the integration of technology in healthcare, optimizing quality, accessibility, and cost-efficiency of care.

Dr. Chaiken's thought leadership is featured in his groundbreaking book *Navigating the Code: How Revolutionary Technology Transforms the Patient-Physician Journey*. This book is the forerunner to his current work, *Future Healthcare 2035: How Artificial Intelligence Transforms the Patient-Physician Journey*, which delves into the transformative potential of artificial intelligence in redefining healthcare delivery and patient care.

At the helm of DocsNetwork Ltd., Dr. Chaiken has provided invaluable guidance to various healthcare organizations, including the National Institutes of Health, the UK National Health Service, and tech giants such as McKesson, Infor, and Salesforce/ Tableau. His consultancy work emphasizes patient safety, clinician technology adoption, and effective healthcare change management, underscoring his expertise in marrying clinical needs with technological advancements.

A celebrated keynote speaker, Dr. Chaiken has captivated audiences worldwide with over 60 CME lectures, sharing his expertise on the pivotal role of technology in healthcare, patient safety, and the future of healthcare artificial intelligence. Moving beyond traditional publication contributions, Dr. Chaiken now engages a broad audience through his biweekly LinkedIn newsletter, "Future-Primed Healthcare," and his "Dr. Barry Speaks" YouTube channel. These platforms showcase his insights on the latest trends and innovations in healthcare, reflecting his commitment to leading the conversation on healthcare's digital transformation.

Dr. Chaiken's academic foundation includes a medical degree from SUNY Downstate Health Sciences University, a Master in Public Health degree from the Harvard School of Public Health, and a Bachelor of Arts in Psychology from the University at Albany. His postgraduate training was completed at the Centers for Disease Control and Prevention as an Epidemic Intelligence Service Officer and at the New Jersey State Department of Health as a preventive medicine resident, highlighting his broad expertise in public health and preventive medicine.

As an Overseas Fellow of the Royal Society of Medicine and a Fellow of the Health Information Management and Systems Society (HIMSS), Dr. Chaiken's career is defined by his professional achievements and resilience as a cancer survivor. This personal journey has deepened his advocacy for patient-centered care, adding a unique perspective to his work on improving healthcare systems.

Beyond his professional endeavors, Dr. Chaiken is deeply committed to shaping the future of healthcare through education. He serves as a guest lecturer at prestigious institutions and contributes to the development of the next generation of healthcare leaders and innovators.

www.ingramcontent.com/pod-product-compliance
Lightning Source LLC
Chambersburg PA
CBHW050238270326
41914CB00034BA/1969/J